The DOCTOR and the WORD

Reginald Cherry, M.D.
with Larry Keefauver

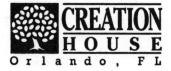
CREATION HOUSE
Orlando, FL

THE DOCTOR AND THE WORD by Reginald Cherry
Published by Creation House
Strang Communications Company
600 Rinehart Road
Lake Mary, Florida 32746
Web site: http://www.creationhouse.com

Copyright © 1996 by Reginald Cherry
All rights reserved
Library of Congress Catalog Card Number: 96-83758
International Standard Book Number: 0-88419-513-9 (pbk)

9012345 BBG 876543
Printed in the United States of America

This book is dedicated to my beloved wife, Linda;
my partner, my nurse, my cohost and
my constant companion.

Thank you, Linda, for praying me into the kingdom
of God and for constantly encouraging me
and strengthening me.

I love you dearly.

Acknowledgments

There is no greater honor on earth than for God to burn a message in your heart to help His people. As this message develops, God uses family and friends to give words of encouragement and godly wisdom to bring these truths from the heart to the written word.

I am deeply grateful to many special people.

To Florence Graves Cherry, my mother, who taught me the love of the written word and encouraged me to study.

To Pastor John Osteen, my pastor, my teacher and my friend, who first encouraged me to write a book.

To Paul and Jan Crouch, who believed in me and allowed me to share God's health laws on the Trinity Broadcasting Network.

To Brother R. W. Schambach, whose love and friendship has seen us through many valleys and placed us on many mountain tops.

To Tommy Burchfield, for his love, support and encouragement over the years and for standing with me as a brother.

To Larry Keefauver and Creation House, for their godly wisdom and endless support in getting God's message published for His people.

To you, the reader, for your love and support over the years. May this book give you answers, hope and encouragement.

Contents

This book is the story of a medical doctor who was changed forever by the touch of the Master Physician. You will see how the simple yet powerful force of God's presence and the flow of the Holy Spirit's response to prayer have changed patients' lives.

This book will take you on a fascinating journey into a modern medical clinic where biblical principles are used to help people receive healing from cancer, heart disease and "all manner of illnesses." I will share concepts which God has shown me that have resulted in healings for people who were caught in modern medicine's so-called impossible situations. These testimonies of healings will astound you, give you hope and increase your faith in the great healing power of the God we serve. It is my prayer that from these pages will flow God's answer to your problem.

— Reginald Cherry, M.D.

Chapter 1

DOCTOR and the WORD

THE WORD CHANGES A MEDICAL PRACTICE

The world surrounding us is filled with advanced technology, the exploration of space and the world of computer information accessible via the internet. Information is increasing so rapidly that we have had to develop highly specialized disciplines just to keep up with the explosion of information.

Medicine is no exception. Medical technology is exploding with tests such as PET scans, MRI scans and laser surgery increasing daily. Our diagnostic clinic in Houston utilizes some of the latest technological advances to conduct our comprehensive medical exams and to diagnose difficult, challenging diseases. Yet with all of today's technology, many patients are increasingly frustrated by enduring multiple medical tests costing thousands of dollars but still revealing no answers to their problems. And often doctors seem as cold and technical as the machines they use to conduct the various tests.

For years I was a Christian physician, practicing medicine in a Christian environment, surrounded by prayer and focused on the power of the Holy Spirit to guide me into all truth. But I was frustrated — some patients were healed supernaturally through faith and the prayer of agreement while God used medicine and His anointing upon medical techniques to achieve healing in others. For a long time this puzzled me.

Then my medical practice was changed forever by a simple scripture written nearly two thousand years ago. I will share this scripture and illustrate its operation in the modern practice of medicine with two unusual examples of healings that I witnessed personally.

As I questioned why some patients were healed one way through a divine touch of God and others were healed through traditional medicine, God showed me a biblical principle. I had read the scripture many times over the years but was unaware it would become the guiding scriptural principle that would lead to healing for thousands of our patients.

Discovering the Pathway to Healing in Scripture

John 9 contains the story of a man who evidently had a congenital form of blindness as he had been blind since birth. But when Jesus passed by this blind man, He performed one of the most unusual healings recorded in the Bible. Jesus mixed clay and saliva and placed it on the eyes of the blind man (John 9:6). But the man was not immediately healed when Jesus touched him. That intrigued me. We often have the image of Jesus healing people supernaturally with an instant manifestation of healing (this was often the case in Jesus' ministry). But I believe this story in John 9 illustrates a principle of healing other than instant manifestation. After Jesus touched the blind man's eyes with clay and saliva, He instructed him to go down a certain path, bend down into a pool (Siloam), place water in his hands and wash his eyes. Then the scripture records that "he went his way therefore, and washed, and came seeing" (v. 7, KJV). The blind man was healed as he obeyed the instructions of Jesus.

This scripture illustrates the healing power of God in a unique way. Through John 9:7 God showed me this principle of healing: Each person must follow a distinctive pathway to healing; that just as the blind man was healed in a unique way, the manifestation of healing will come to each one of us in a unique way.

The ramifications of this principle are far-reaching. For many the pathway to healing is a supernatural one where God instructs us to simply believe through faith for our healing, and as a result, the manifestation will come. For some the supernatural manifestation may come as they are anointed with oil in a healing service. Others may be led simply to speak to their disease for healing to be manifested. Yet for others the pathway to healing lies through God's anointing on a natural substance — something we can touch, see, hold and experience through our senses. In other words, God's anointing may rest on the use of traditional medicine, a plant, an herb, a surgical procedure and so on — just as the healing anointing of God flowed through mud and saliva as Jesus touched the blind man in John 9. As we seek God for the unique pathway to our healing, we too will realize total and complete healing.

The revelation contained in this scripture has changed the way we pray for patients at our clinic. We continue to look to God as our Healer through the completed work of Jesus on Calvary two thousand years ago. Prayer is the central focus of getting our patients healed. But because of John 9:7, I am now praying a different way than I used to pray and encouraging my patients to do the same. The results, which I will share with you shortly, are dramatic.

Go to the Father in the name of Jesus, seeking His specific pathway to your healing.

As you pray this way, you are not limiting God's healing flow. God's pathway for your healing may be a supernatural, miraculous touch from Him. On the other hand, there may be a series of steps that God wants you to follow just as Jesus told the blind man to follow specific guidelines to achieve his healing. Praying this way opens a new dimension to God's healing manifestation in your body.

Dramatic Results in Our Medical Practice

We use this seeking principle daily in our medical practice. Let me share with you two dramatic healings that took place as a result of praying and seeking God specifically for an individual's pathway to healing.

I will never forget one lady who came for a complete medical evaluation. She had no symptoms in her body but sought an examination simply because she wanted to keep her temple strong and uncover any early attacks that might be taking place against her body. We had nearly finished her morning of testing when suddenly I noticed a large polyp, or growth, in her lower colon during the colon examination.

Usually God leads us to have such polyps removed in an early stage to prevent the potential development of colon cancer. However, God stopped me and told me that we were not to remove this lady's polyp surgically. I completed the exam and left the lady so my staff could complete the rest of her tests. I quickly went into my office and shut the door. I sat at my desk and prayed, "God, this lady has a definite growth in her colon. This could cause serious problems for her."

All doctors are taught in medical school that polyps of this nature must be removed. This is the approach that is almost always used in modern medicine. Suddenly God was telling me to do something that went against everything I was taught in medical school. I did not want to miss God on this one because it could have been a matter of life and death for this sweet Christian lady. On the other hand, God spoke to me as clearly as I have ever heard Him speak that she was not to have surgery. So I told God that I did not understand what He was doing. But if He did not want the polyp surgically removed, I asked God please to tell me what to do next. I certainly did not know what He had in mind.

God answered my prayer by saying, "Bring the lady into your office after her tests are completed. Explain what you found in her colon, and have her agree with you in prayer that the polyp will be healed and will disappear. Instruct the lady to come back in thirty days to have her colon checked again." God had revealed to me this patient's unique pathway to healing.

I had broken out in a mild sweat because of the responsibility of making this decision. Yet I knew what God had told me. Regardless of what all of my professors in medical school had said, I decided in faith that I was going to do it God's way. As instructed, I brought the lady into my office. She was a strong Christian lady, a woman of great faith who obviously walked closely with the Lord. I explained to her that there was a growth in her colon and that we usually remove such growths surgically, but God had told me to do otherwise in her situation. I told her that God instructed us to agree in prayer for her healing and that she would see the manifestation of healing without surgery. I

11

asked, "Are you willing to pray and agree with me for your healing?"

"Doctor," she said, "let's quit this talking and start praying now." So I grabbed her hands, and we prayed the prayer of agreement as God had instructed. We agreed that the polyp would disappear. At the conclusion of our prayer, God gave me one final instruction for her. I asked her to come back to the clinic in four weeks to recheck that area. God is not a God of foolishness. God wanted to confirm His word with physical evidence of healing. The woman readily agreed, and she left my office.

Four weeks later she returned to the clinic. In her chart I had marked the exact location of the polyp in centimeters. I again examined her colon. At the precise location of the previously noted growth, I could find no evidence of an abnormality. Her colon was as smooth and normal as it could be.

You may wonder why God chose to heal her this way. Perhaps she would have suffered a complication when the surgical procedure was done. Perhaps a blood vessel could have been ruptured causing her to bleed profusely. Sometimes a small tear or perforation can take place in the wall of the colon during surgery. We can never know all these things, but we do know that her body was "fearfully and wonderfully made" by her Creator (Ps. 139:14, NIV). By being open to God's specific pathway of healing, we saw a miracle take place.

A second illustration of God's supernatural healing further demonstrates the principle that there is a unique pathway of healing for each individual. This is one of the more unusual medical cases I have encountered.

A lady who lived in the northern mountain states flew to our clinic in Houston after seeing five or six specialists because of an intense rash on both of her hands. Like the woman with the issue of blood, she had spent all her living upon physicians and could not be healed of any (Luke 8:43).

When I did her examination I could hardly believe my eyes. I had never seen anything like it. She had a condition medically know as nummular eczematous dermatitis. I guess the best way to describe it would be leprosy of the hands. Her hands were cracked, crusty and bleeding on both sides, and there was not a smooth area anywhere. As she sat in my office the tears ran down her cheeks when she described the torment this affliction had brought to her. She was a sweet Christian lady but was embarrassed to be around people or even to go to church because of her hands. She wore gloves to hide her embarrassment all the time, even in hot summer weather. Doctors had tried everything else — but nothing had worked.

As I finished the various tests I went into my office, closed the door and began to pray. "God, I have never seen anything like this in my life. This poor lady has suffered so much and spent so much money trying to get cured. Now she has come all these miles, looking to me for the solution to her healing."

God quickly pointed out that she came to Houston not so much to see me but to seek Him together with me for healing in her body. I prayed according to the John 9:7 principle. In the name of Jesus I asked God to show me the pathway for this lady's healing. I wanted to lay hands on her and see her instantly supernaturally healed. God's pathway, however, was different. As I prayed at my desk prior to talking to this lady, God took me back some twenty-five years to medical school to a one-hour lecture by a dermatologist (skin specialist). I had not thought of this lecture in years. The professor said that he once had a patient with a severe eruption on the skin. He mentioned using a certain type of anti-inflammatory cream but discovered that the cream had to be covered with an occlusive dressing.

Suddenly God showed me that this was the answer to the problems this lady was having with her hands.

I called her into the office, and she sat down in front of my desk. I told her I was sorry she had to wait so long but that I was praying about her condition. I told her that God gave me the answer for her healing. As I saw her eyes well up with tears, mine did the same.

She wasn't prepared for what I was getting ready to tell her. God had instructed me to use a cream, but He told me that the reason she was not healing was that the cream was not being absorbed. He then told me to have her use plastic wrap each evening after she applied the cream. I took out my prescription pad, wrote down the name of a certain prescription and gave it to her. I then took out a second prescription and wrote out the instructions on how to use the cream and gave it to her. The look on her face defied words. She looked at me as if to say, "Surely you are kidding me, Dr. Cherry."

I explained the procedure to her, asking her to go to the pharmacy, get the prescription and then go to the grocery store and get plastic wrap.

"If you will follow this plan," I told her, "your hands will be healed." The look on her face must have been similar to the blind man's face when Jesus performed the unusual healing of putting mud and saliva on his eyes. She did not argue with me or begin questioning me but simply said, "I will do as you say, Dr. Cherry." We had a prayer together, and she went her way.

I had forgotten her case until a year later when she walked into my office for an annual examination. As I reviewed her history she did not say a word but simply held out her hands, turning them over several times. Her hands were as smooth and tender as a baby's. Suddenly the tears began rolling down her cheeks. As I looked at her hands and looked into her eyes, God brought to my remembrance the woman with the leprosy-like affliction on her hands.

I remembered the instructions God had given me a year ago for her healing. The tears ran down my cheeks as we sat in amazement at the awesome healing power of God.

These two healings demonstrate the unique healing power of God. I have seen hundreds of patients healed as we sought God together for their unique pathway to healing according to John 9:7. Many were healed with no traditional medicine whatsoever just like the woman with the polyp; for others the healing anointing was manifested through common physical substances, and in some cases these were most unusual.

Praying according to John 9:7 opens a new dimension to God's healing power. It does not limit us, and it does not limit God. His Word reveals that with the stripes of Jesus we have already been healed (Is. 53:5). You may have yet to see a manifestation of healing in your body. A new hope will enter your spirit as you read these principles from the heart of your Father. Yes, we would all like to be healed instantly, supernaturally and miraculously. Thank God that miracles are still taking place. Seek God for the specific pathway He has determined for your healing. Realize that your pathway to healing may involve the use of certain natural substances.

One of Satan's most effective ways to stop you and keep you from finishing the race to which God has called you is to attack your temple — your physical body. Applying this principle from John 9 will lead you to the pathway to your healing.

An important part of the completed manifestation of your healing is finding a doctor who understands this principle and will pray in agreement with you. I could never help patients find their pathway to healing without prayer. Many times God works through the technology of medicine. As a Spirit-led doctor hears from God and turns to the unique pathway that God has chosen for a patient's healing, he will know when and how to use modern technology or when to back away from technology to allow God to heal supernaturally.

The practice of modern medicine which is bathed in prayer and guided by the Holy Spirit is one of the most exciting endeavors a human being can undertake. However, my journey to this exciting God-centered medical practice was a long one. It took me many years to understand the principles of healing and how they could be incorporated in medicine today. And it all began with that wonderful, unusual and revelatory passage in John 9.

I invite you to join me in discovering God's healing covenant and His healing promises for:

- Finding your pathway of healing

- Hindrances to healing that you can avoid

- Applying your authority and power over sickness and disease

- Using natural ways God provided to prevent, protect and heal from major killers such as heart disease, cancer and diabetes

No matter what your problem or illness, God has a pathway for that manifestation of healing to take place. This book will help you to find new hope for your healing. Your faith will be increased as you read these pages and understand God's pathway of healing for you.

Chapter 2

DOCTOR and the WORD

THE POWER OF GOD CHANGES A DOCTOR

To understand this book you should understand a bit about me. How I became a doctor and what God did in my life has shaped *The Doctor and the Word*. As I tell my story, I want you to remember this testimony is not just about Dr. Cherry. I tell it to show what God did in my life — a life that now belongs to Christ. Here's my story just as it happened.

Humble Beginnings — But a Rich Dream

The first six years of my life were lived in the dusty, rural town of Mansfield in the Ouachita Mountains in the hills of western Arkansas. The town is north of Poteau Mountain and east of Sugarloaf Mountain; west of Abbott and east of

Hartford. For generations my entire family had lived and died in those hills of western Arkansas. From my earliest recollections, I wanted to be a doctor. I do not have the foggiest idea how such an impossible dream entered the head of a boy who grew up in the mountains, but that was my goal — to be a doctor!

Who Was Billy Graham?

Our home in that little Arkansas town stood right across the street from the Methodist church. But God was not a major focus in our home. My parents occasionally took me to Sunday school, church services or to vacation Bible school in the summer, but our lives were not centered on God.

When I was six, we left Mansfield and moved to the big city of Little Rock. Dad worked as a salesman for a meat company, and that meant we moved often. We soon transferred to Oklahoma City and finally ended up in Texas, where I grew up from my elementary years into being a teenager.

From the time I was in the third or fourth grade, I was repeatedly drawn to a television program with a preacher by the name of Billy Graham. I could never explain my attraction, but when Billy Graham came on television, I would get a notebook and take notes even as a very young boy. I wrote down almost everything he said as well as all the scriptures he used. Then I would study those notes and read the Bible verses for a month or two. I would gradually put them aside and forget them. Nothing happened inside of me even though my curiosity about what Billy Graham was saying would stir me. This happened over and over again throughout the years. I watched the newspapers to find out when he was scheduled to be on television. I was drawn to him and to his message. Even though God was not a dominating force in my family's life, the Lord was already pulling me to Him at an early age. But those early encounters with God would not take root in my life until years later.

Be a Doctor? Impossible!

I desperately wanted to become a physician, but there was little money for my schooling. College, much less medical school, seemed far beyond my reach. But I did know how to take one step toward my impossible dream — I knew how to study! I believed that if I had the necessary grades I could overcome the lack of money. So I studied very, very hard. When it came time to apply to college, I began looking at various Texas schools. One school in particular drew me like a magnet — Baylor University.

God was at work in my life behind the scenes. The impossible became possible. I received a scholarship to Baylor. At that time, I thought my good grades and scholarships made it possible to go through premed school. God was orchestrating a plan that I would not understand until later.

Trying to Make the Grade

Baylor University was the largest Baptist university in the world. I knew I had to make high grades in order to proceed with my goal of going to medical school. Only the students with the highest grades could ever make it to medical school.

All the premed students would sit in the back of our Old Testament classes and make bets with each other as to who was going to make the highest grade on the final exam. Can you imagine doing that in an Old Testament class? We memorized almost the whole Old Testament. I knew the Adamic Covenant, the Noahic Covenant and the Levitic Covenant. I could tell you about every covenant God made with His people — from the old to the new. We would see who could make the highest grade above one hundred on the final exam. (If you answered the bonus questions, you could go above one hundred points.) At one point I even lost a bet for forgetting some of the genealogy of Enoch. It's disconcerting to me now to think that we approached the Old Testament as though it were a physics or chemistry class.

In our New Testament class the professors wrote on the chalkboard about the blood of Jesus. We got out our notebooks and wrote, "the blood of Jesus is the atonement for our sins." They talked about redemption, sanctification, justification and propitiation. I knew it all and could write a ten-page paper about any one of these subjects for a test. But I was as lost as a road lizard going nowhere. After final exams were over I forgot everything I knew about the Old and New Testaments. Although I was learning the awesome truths about salvation in Jesus Christ, my only concerns were good grades, medical school and winning the class bets!

As if studying all those biblical courses to get through Baylor was not enough, it was a big aggravation to me that chapel was required — we had to attend chapel for two hours every week during the first two years at Baylor. If we skipped chapel too many times, we had to write a twenty-page term paper on some aspect of religion. So I went to chapel until I devised a plan to skip it without being caught. Those individuals in charge of chapel services did not really care who sat in the chapel seats — they just wanted the seats full. So we would seek out somebody who had already put in his chapel time and pay him to sit in our chapel seats.

It is hard for me to confess such things now. I now drive forty-five miles several times a week, every week, to go to my church for worship and Bible study. But in my college days before I knew the Lord, I worked so hard to get out of chapel just two times a week. After I met the Lord, being in His presence was so wonderful I could not get enough "chapel" time with Him. (I am sure you feel that way as well.)

Only a Few Realize Their Dreams

During my first day of campus orientation at Baylor I sat in a fifteen hundred-seat auditorium filled with premed students as a professor announced, "I want you to look around at all of the students in this room. Four years from now only twenty of you will be going to medical school!" That's not the best news to hear when starting off a medical career. In fact, it's downright discouraging. That professor made another statement that stuck in my mind. He said, "The twenty that are selected will be determined primarily by how hard they study and how high their grade point average is."

Now, I knew how to study. Once again I began to trust my abilities to accomplish what only God could do. The time would come when I would face an impossible situation that I could not handle. I could delay the inevitable but could never avoid it. One day my dreams would have to be surrendered to the only One who could do the impossible. For the moment, I pressed blindly on toward my dream — medical school.

Maintaining a high grade point average in premed was very frustrating. One day while in my third year at Baylor, I was looking through a brochure when I found out that certain selected students with high enough grade point averages could leave Baylor after three years of study and go straight to medical school. I thought, *Now that's the best news I have heard.* Immediately, without telling a soul, I filled out applications to several medical schools, never dreaming I would be accepted. Surprise! Several schools accepted me. I rushed to a phone and called home.

I was the first child among all my relatives to graduate from college. No one from our family had ever finished college. I called my mother, blurting out my news: "Mama, I'm not going to graduate from Baylor."

Hurt saturated her voice, "Honey, you're what? Why not?"

"Well," I continued, "I'm going on to medical school. They let me in after three years. They didn't want me around here anymore, I guess."

So I left Baylor and headed for medical school.

The Godless Void at Medical School

Medical school is probably the most godless environment that I have ever been in. I felt no touch of God directly in my life while I was in medical school. This is ironic, because medical school was the very place where I was studying the body, the temple of the Holy Spirit (1 Cor. 3:16-17). I studied and learned about God's temple without ever knowing who created it. We only addressed the physical and mental aspects of man.

Spiritual things were often viewed as abnormalities. In fact, when born-again, Christian patients told us that God had spoken to them we sent them for a psychiatric consultation in order to make sure they did not have early symptoms of schizophrenia or some kind of mental disturbance. That's the way religion was viewed by professors and doctors.

After graduating from medical school my next step was to specialize in cardiology and internal medicine.

Preventive Medicine — A Unique Opportunity

It wasn't long before a unique opportunity presented itself. I met a physician named Dr. Kenneth Cooper. Dr. Cooper practiced an unusual kind of medicine called preventive medicine (at least at that time it was unusual). This appealed to me. I had always had a little bit different approach to medicine than most doctors who were trained to treat disease and illness. For some reason I simply was not happy or satisfied with just waiting until a person got sick enough to treat him. I wanted to prevent disease as well as treat it.

So when I heard of an opportunity to get involved with preventive medicine, I grasped the baton and decided to meet with Dr. Cooper. I declared to him, "I would like to come to work for you." It did not matter to me that I was just twenty-six years old and other doctors who were forty and fifty years old had also applied for a position at Dr. Cooper's prestigious clinic.

It just so happened that they were in urgent need for a doctor. They had a sudden vacancy and needed a physician to see previously scheduled patients at the clinic immediately. So Dr. Cooper said, "Come out, and let me talk to you."

During my initial visit, Dr. Cooper offered, "Well, we will hire you."

So I joined the staff of one of the country's most elite clinics, The Aerobic Center/Cooper Clinic in Dallas, Texas. Patients began calling and asking to see me because their friends had been seen by me. Soon my name got to be well-known among a small group of people as I began practicing preventive medicine with nutrition, exercise and comprehensive lifestyle changes.

My pride began to grow as an inner longing inside of me desired to be fulfilled. I began making money in amounts I had never dreamed of making. I was asked often to give speeches. Patients asked for me by name. A dark, inner self-centeredness began to grow, reaching out and filling the void within. I became very arrogant and decided to leave the clinic. I will never forget the day I went into Dr. Cooper's office and said, "Dr. Cooper, I'm going to need to be moving on."

Surprised, he asked, "What do you mean?"

I said, "Well, I've worked here for you a year, and I appreciate what you've done for me. But, Dr. Cooper, Dallas is just not big enough for both of us." Here I was in my twenties, an insignificant doctor, confronting a man who had written a best-selling book with over six million copies in print. He had spoken all over the world and was the leading figure in preventive medicine. He smiled weakly at me and said, "You are making a mistake, Reg. You are making a mistake. If you'll stay here, I'll make you the clinic director."

"No," I said, "I've made up my mind. I've got to go on, got to leave here."

He told me, "You'll never make it."

But I said, "Well, I'm going to make it. I'm going to Houston because there's not a preventive medical practice there, and I'm going to start my own clinic."

"You'll never make it," Dr. Cooper told me. "We've had other doctors leave here saying the same thing, but they haven't made it."

But I still protested, "Not me, Dr. Cooper."

Even though Dr. Cooper was a strong, decent Christian man, I waved good-bye and headed for Houston. I thought, *Man, I know it all. I've worked under him, and I'm going to pass him up.* It was with that arrogance inside of me that I arrived in Houston.

God deals with pride like that.

We can never come to know God intimately without being broken.

I had not yet been broken, but the time of His reckoning with me was coming.

On My Own in Houston

It was the midseventies when I arrived in Houston and opened a clinic in a northern suburb in Montgomery County. I was determined to have a big beautiful clinic and make a lot of money. That first year I nearly starved to death! There were very few people willing to drive out to Montgomery County in 1975 to see a doctor practicing some kind of medicine they had never even heard of before. It was rough. I decided that I needed to get closer to town, so I moved my office to the middle part of Houston.

Having discovered that I had worked with Dr. Cooper, a reporter for the *Houston Post* newspaper called me up one day and said, "Dr. Cherry, I want to do an article about preventive medicine." She explained that no doctor at that time in Houston was practicing preventive medicine since it was such a new specialty, and she was intrigued.

She interviewed me at the office and wrote an article about my clinic. My practice started growing. Business increased. Soon large companies were signing up their employees to come through the clinic for diagnostic and physical examinations. Company presidents, important executives and wealthy professionals from all over came in for physicals. The clinic became a very busy place. I realized that we were going to have to expand and hire more doctors because I could not handle it all by myself. So we started looking for opportunities to expand our facility and hire other doctors.

At that time a forty-million-dollar fitness facility was opening in Houston. It cost ten thousand dollars to join the club. I said to my staff, "You know, I need to be part of this because this is where all the action is. Look at all the space they have on the West Loop in Houston. We need to be over there. Jogging trails, tennis courts and other facilities will all be readily available."

So I went over to this exclusive club and rented clinic space. Our business started to grow there and become very successful. We had to hire two additional doctors. I started getting calls from all parts of the country to make speeches on preventive medicine. It was a new specialty in medicine and companies wanted to hear about it. Professional groups wanted to know how they could prevent heart disease, cancer and other stress or diet-related illnesses. My ego was building and building.

I was flown to Lake Tahoe, flown to Florida — I was flown all over the country making speeches, writing articles, doing all that I had ever dreamed of and more. All the while I was becoming more and more arrogant.

My success was feeding desires I never knew I had. At the age of twenty-eight, money, possessions, recognition, power and prestige were all coming my way. All of those things that I longed for — the reputation I wanted, the name I wanted, the wealth I wanted — were all at my fingertips. Doctors were actually working for me. I began looking around to see how I could spend the money I was making.

Realizing My Dream but Still Longing for More

Money became the driving force in my life. I thought money was the thing that would compensate for what I had never had as a child. Looking back now, I realize that Jesus was right when He said, "No one can serve two masters. Either he will hate the one and love the other, or he will be devoted to the one and despise the other. You cannot serve both God and Money" (Matt. 6:24, NIV).

Money became my master. I never had much money as a child. Now I had it — or rather, it had me. I started buying things. I bought property in the county where I lived and more property back in Arkansas where I used to live. Soon buying land became boring, so I started looking around for other things to buy.

One day I decided that what I needed was a fleet of automobiles — one of every kind of vehicle available. I bought a family sedan, a sports car, a pickup truck and a four-wheel drive vehicle for when it rained and the roads became slippery. I enjoyed lining up all of those vehicles just like a fleet. When one of them got a bit dirty or low on gasoline I simply used another vehicle from my fleet. But I became bored with the vehicles and looked around for something else.

One day as I was driving down the road I saw a bulldozer, and thought, *Now this is what I need — a bulldozer.* I went down to the dealer and bought it too, a great big bulldozer. I had no inkling of how to operate a bulldozer, but the man that sold it to me was smart. He said, "Dr. Cherry, I don't know what you intend to use this for, but you need to put a rack on it."

I soon discovered why he wanted me to buy a rack for the front of my bulldozer. It became an indispensable device as I started uprooting trees on a piece of property that I owned. I removed stumps and pushed rocks and dirt and other things all over with that bulldozer. I wasn't very careful in the way I operated the machine, and tree limbs bounced off the top and sides. I nearly tore up the machine *and* me in the process. It doesn't take a lot of knowledge to operate a bulldozer. The latest models are fully automatic; you just put it in gear and shove the lever forward. Once moving, there is not much that will slow down a bulldozer.

However, I did find a few things that would stop a bulldozer. One time I drove the bulldozer onto the top of a stump. The tracks were suspended in the air turning around and around. The most embarrassing thing in the world is having to call a heavy-duty wrecker to pull a bulldozer off a stump. To this day, I cringe just remembering the smirk on the face of the wrecker's driver when he came to pull me off that stump.

Eventually even the bulldozer became boring. Where could I turn next to satisfy the longing that had developed within? Where does one go from a bulldozer? What's next — a crane or an earthmover? What was left for me to buy?

Vehicles no longer filled the void. But I remained a driven person, doing everything I did at full steam ahead. I decided to take up long-distance running, determining to become the best runner there ever was. I took up marathon running. While there isn't anything wrong with marathon running, I worshiped it. After spending the mornings at my clinic seeing my patients, every afternoon I went to Memorial Park in Houston where I would run, sometimes twenty miles at a time. Can you imagine lapping a trail time and time again, spending hours just running in circles? For a while this satisfied me as people patted me on the back for my efforts. But in time my knees became so achy and sore that I thought I would never be able to exercise or even take another step again.

I was living much the way Solomon did as seen in Ecclesiastes. He tried to find meaning in every pursuit of life — wealth, education, pleasure, work and fame. Nothing filled his emptiness, and he finally admitted, "Meaningless! Meaningless!...Everything is meaningless!" (Eccl. 12:8, NIV).

Speed and fast cars became an obsession with me. I developed a perfect alibi for going fast. When I wanted to go fast I wouldn't wear a suit or a sports coat. I would put on my white physician's coat, get in my little sports car and speed down the freeway. If a policeman stopped me, I got out of the car and said, "I have an emergency, Officer. I have to get down to the clinic fast."

Of course the officer would respond, "No problem, Doctor, go on. But be careful." I'm telling you, I had more emergencies than any doctor in Houston! And I had a preventive medicine practice! I was driven — looking for something, anything, to satisfy the longing in my life.

My clinic was prospering. However, I became somewhat of a tyrant as a boss. Preventive medicine was so popular that we were deluged with applications of people who wanted to work for us. Doctors from all over the country were applying for a position at our clinic. Nurses and technicians lined up for openings. If employees did not do what I wanted, I would fire them, pull out another application and hire someone else. It was no big deal to me. In fact, I prided myself on how quickly I got rid of people who were not measuring up to my impossible standards. I was driven and miserable. I drove my staff as hard and fast as I drove my sports car — and made them just as miserable as I was myself.

Facing My Emptiness

One day I walked into the clinic and did not think the staff was hustling fast enough. So I instructed one of the technicians to buy two tapes to play on our music system in the clinic. I told him, "Every morning when I walk in I want the soundtracks from *Rocky* and *Patton* to be playing, and I want the staff to get some hustle to them."

He looked at me in astonishment and said, "You want the tapes played every day?"

I said, "Every day."

I thought faster music would motivate my staff. I wanted to get them moving faster. Patients loved it. But the staff thought I was weird (to say the least). I was miserable inside! I had inner turmoil and a raging drive within me all the time. I never smiled when I was at the clinic. I was always dead serious — trying to drive and push everything and everyone, including myself, harder and faster. Why did I push so hard? For prestige, fame, power and money!

A drama began to unfold at that time in the clinic. There was a noticeable change in the life of one of my nurses. I saw something different about her and heard a rumor that she had accepted Jesus. She became one of those Jesus people. She "found religion."

At first, I didn't pay too much attention to it. But one day as she looked at the situation in my life, she saw my misery and the longing that I had deep within. She decided that she would start praying for me. Not much happened on the surface except that I kept getting meaner and meaner. One day one of my fleet of vehicles broke down, and I could not get another vehicle delivered to me. I needed a ride to get my car repaired. So I asked this nurse, "On your lunch hour can you run me over to the repair shop to get my car fixed?"

She agreed. As we walked down to the parking garage and approached her car I noticed the small Jesus sticker on the back bumper. I just shook my head. When she started the car, the radio was playing music from a Christian station. I asked, "Do you listen to Christian music?"

She said, "Yes, I listen to Christian music."

I said, "You mean that you listen to hymns all the time?" The only kind of Christian music I knew was "The Old Rugged Cross" and "When the Roll Is Called Up Yonder." She said, "Well, they are not really hymns, but...I'll turn it off."

I started thinking about how different her life seemed to be from my own life. I knew she had lived through a tremendous number of battles and tragedies in her personal life. Yet there was a peace about her, a total change that had occurred within her life. It was obvious to me and to everyone around the clinic.

I found out later that when she decided to start praying for me, she did not pray for me by herself. Instead, she got her whole church to pray for Dr. Cherry. She not only requested prayer for me during her church services but also got her Saturday night prayer group praying by saying, "Will you pray for my mean boss, Dr. Cherry? He needs help. He needs the Lord."

Well, when people start praying, something is going to happen; events and circumstances start changing as God acts. At first, there were no obvious changes in my life. But all those Christians continued to pray for me.

The office circumstances were so deplorable that this nurse decided to leave the clinic. Although she continued to pray for me, she felt that she needed to get out of the clinic. She went to numerous job interviews, but somehow nothing worked out even though she was very qualified. She told herself to hang on in our office a little longer. She kept praying, and her church kept praying. But I was still miserable.

I had reached the end of what satisfaction my money could buy. I had all the prestige, all the patients and all the things that money could buy, but I was still empty within. I was searching; something was missing in my life. And that persistent nurse kept praying and kept praying.

A very subtle change began to occur within me. Suddenly I found myself thinking about God. At first, that's all that was happening. Nothing changed on the outside. But thoughts about God came at the strangest times. God reminded me of the Billy Graham crusades. I even thought back to the time when Billy Graham had come to our town, and I had gone forward to be saved. I remembered all the words I had said as I confessed my faith in Jesus. But they were just words from my lips, not from my heart. I thought back to my days at Baylor University when I had Old and New Testament classes. Words like *redemption* and *sanctification* drifted through my mind. I thought about God more and more frequently.

One day God began to speak to me! He knew I was miserable. The clinic staff knew I was miserable. Everyone saw my turmoil. God said, "I see your misery. I see your seeking. I know about your longings. I see you hungering for something in your life." God knows what we are feeling and thinking even before we express it. "Before a word is on my tongue you know it completely, O Lord" (Ps. 139:4, NIV). He knows what you and I are going through even before we know Him.

I knew that my life was reaching a climax, a crisis point. I knew I needed to make a decision about God. I needed to do something about my frequent thoughts about God — either cast Him totally out of my mind or turn my life over to Him. I was miserable because of all the thoughts about God that I continued having.

Again God spoke to me, "The peace that you want I will give you. That longing in your heart I will satisfy. I will give you the desires of your heart. I will give you total joy and peace in your life."

God was not saying anything to me that He does not say to anyone who is honestly seeking and searching for meaning in life. God promises, "You will seek me and find me when you seek me with your heart" (Jer. 29:13, NIV).

God said, "But there is one thing I ask of you. You must give your whole life to Me. You must give everything in your life to Me." Much like the rich young man in the tenth chapter of Mark, I was confronted with the same decision, "'One thing you lack,' he [Jesus] said. 'Go, sell everything you have and give to the poor, and you will have treasure in heaven. Then come, follow me'" (Mark 10:21, NIV).

I pondered His words. *I don't know about all this*, I thought. *What is He asking? I have a million-dollar medical practice...land...all these cars. Does this mean giving all this to God? I don't know about this.*

God said, "I'll give you the peace that you seek. I'll give you joy unspeakable if you'll give it all to Me, everything you've got." For the first time I was hearing that wonderful promise from God in 1 Peter 1:8-9, "Though you have not seen him [the Lord], you love him; and even though you do not see him now, you believe in him and are filled with an inexpressible and glorious joy, for you are receiving the goal of your faith, the salvation of your souls" (NIV).

God said one final thing that left me speechless. "You have been to this point before with Me. I remember when you watched Billy Graham and decided to live for Me, but it quickly slipped away. I remember when you said those words accepting Jesus as your Savior, but you only said them with your mouth, not with your heart. This is the last time I'm going to bother you about serving Me." I felt as if this would be my last chance to accept Christ totally and give my life to Him.

I was paralyzed. Somehow all my life I had told myself, "There's always tomorrow. I'll serve God tomorrow, but today is for me." Suddenly there would be no tomorrow. I knew this was my last opportunity with God, and I was terrified at the thought.

I will never forget that night in late November of 1979 when I called out to God and said, "God, I have no idea what I'm doing." Then without knowing what I was saying, I said the name Jesus for the first time in years. "Jesus, I give You everything I own. I'm sorry for the life I've lived. I want to live for You the rest of my days. I give You my life."

It might not have been a precise, scriptural prayer, but as soon as I said those words I knew I was a new person. From that moment, Dr. Cherry was born-again!

Beginning a New Life!

I didn't know what I was doing, but I knew that something inside of me was totally different. I had a joy that I had never felt before. I was born-again! I was a new creation. I started to experience what Paul wrote about, "Therefore, if anyone is in Christ, he is a new creation; the old has gone, the new has come!" (2 Cor. 5:17, NIV).

But I was such a baby. I was just like a blank wall ready

to be written on by God's hand. My first thought was to sell my medical practice and go to Africa as a missionary. Somehow I just knew that becoming a missionary was what a real Christian doctor would do.

God began speaking to me. "Did I say anything to you about going to Africa and becoming a missionary?"

"Well, no, God," I answered. "But I know that's what You want me to do."

But God said, "Stay right where you are. I'm going to use you right where you are."

Well that was good news to me! I didn't really want to go to Africa; but I was willing, and God saw my heart. One day I looked at my snazzy sports car and thought, *I'm going down and sell that sports car. I'm going to buy a Volkswagen because I know a real Christian wouldn't drive a snazzy sports car.* I meant what I said and was on my way to do it. Even though the sports car was paid for, I thought I had to buy a Volkswagen to be holy. As I drove, I said to God, "God, I love this sports car."

Again God spoke to me, "Did I tell you to sell your car and buy a Volkswagen?"

"Well, no, God," I answered once again. "But I know You wouldn't want me driving a sports car."

"Don't sell your car," God responded. "Keep your car."

Things were sounding better and better to me all the time. Being born-again was pretty good after all. When I walked into the clinic the day after I was saved, everyone seemed to know that something had happened to me. I called the nurse that had been praying for me into my office before we started seeing patients. When she came in I was standing by my bookcase with a smile on my face. I looked at her and said, "I found God." (As a baby Christian that's all I knew to say.)

She said, "You...you what?"

"I found God," I said again. She could not believe it.

Although she had been praying for me for months she could not believe God had answered her prayers. She could not help noticing how different I looked, though.

She said, "You accepted Jesus as your Lord? You said the sinner's prayer? You are born-again?"

I answered, "Yes, I've done all that."

When I went home that night something she had said began to bother me. That morning she had asked, "Did you say the sinner's prayer?"

What's the sinner's prayer? I thought to myself. *I have never heard of that.*

I thought the sinner's prayer was a specific prayer in the Bible like the Lord's prayer. So I began searching in my Bible that night trying to look up the sinner's prayer in the concordance. I could not find it anywhere. That bothered me, so at work the next day I called her back into my office and said, "I can't find the sinner's prayer in the Bible."

She said, "Did you confess your sins to Jesus?"

I said, "Oh, yes, I did that."

"Well," she continued, "did you accept Him into your heart and make Him part of your life?"

"Oh, yes, I did all that."

Then she said, "You've said the sinner's prayer. That's all you have to do. You've already done it. You've been born again!"

Was I relieved! "That's good, because I worried about it all night last night," I confessed as she tried to disguise a grin.

That nurse who prayed for her mean boss and tried to quit her job at the clinic several times was Linda, who is now my wife. She is still a part-time nurse and, together with me, raised our two children. Linda is my cohost on our weekly television program, *The Doctor and the Word,* aired on Trinity Broadcasting Network.

At work, my staff and patients could tell the difference in me. Imagine the situation at my clinic where, before my conversion, I had a great proclivity for firing employees who did not agree with the way I insisted things should be done. Seventeen people worked for me. Now I started hearing them talking amongst themselves and saying, "If we do not find religion, he's going to fire every one of us." These people knew how many applications I had for people wanting to work there — and they were scared!

Two days after I was saved I pushed aside everything on my desk and placed my Bible right on the side of the desk. I didn't care who saw it. I talked about Jesus to anybody, anywhere, anytime. For the first time, I was so joyful and happy. Still my staff wondered what was going to happen next now that I had become a Christian.

The doctors who worked for me were the most concerned about their futures. In my files I had several applications from doctors who wanted to get into preventive medicine. I will never forget one doctor with whom I had had several confrontations. He knew his number was just about up for termination and was very worried. He saw the Bible lying there on my desk, and thought, *Man, I've got to do something to impress him, or Dr. Cherry is going to fire me for sure.* So he went home and got his Bible, brought it to the office and put it on the corner of his desk. When I saw his Bible on his desk, I couldn't believe it!

If you put a Bible on your desk, you must be ready to back it up. He began to get into more hot water than he could have imagined. Christian patients came to see him and saw his Bible on the desk and started talking about Jesus. "Oh, Doctor, I see that you are a Christian. Let me tell you what Jesus did for me. When did you accept Jesus?"

He tried to reply in proper religious terms, "I was baptized as a child in such and such church." But the patients' questions made him so nervous that after two days the Bible had disappeared from his desk.

The panic over my accepting Jesus swept throughout the

clinic. I had peace, joy and happiness in Jesus that I had never experienced before. It poured out of me. But I felt sorry for the other doctors.

One afternoon they came to me and said, "Dr. Cherry, can we set up a time when we can talk to you?" I used to require the doctors on my staff to make an appointment with my secretary to see me even though their offices were right next door to mine.

Now I said, "Sure, come on in, sit down, and let's talk." That threw them off guard immediately because they were not used to being able to approach me. They were as serious as they could be as I said, "What can I do for you?"

Wearily, one doctor commented, "Well, we have been observing your behavior, Dr. Cherry."

I said, "Oh, have you seen the change in me?"

"Yes," one of them responded. "We have seen a change, and we think we have it diagnosed."

"Oh?" I said.

"We've talked extensively about it, and we feel that you have a case of manic-depressive illness and that you are experiencing the manic phase which has made you feel so happy." They didn't realize it, but one of my best subjects in medical school was psychiatry. I don't know why, but I did better in psychiatry than almost any other subject. I knew exactly what manic-depressive illness was. So I looked at them and said, "Well, let me ask you a few questions. Do I show any delusions of grandiosity? Do I show any flight of ideas? Do I show any hyperactivity?"

"Well, no," they said. "You really don't."

After some discussion it was finally obvious to them that there was nothing wrong with my mental faculties and that something had changed inside me. So I said, "Well, I appreciate you boys coming in and sharing that with me, but I think you missed the diagnosis."

So they left. They thought that the clinic would go downhill.

They thought when the word got out that I had become a Jesus man or religious freak, our business would disappear. Yet our business kept booming and growing.

Because of some serious difficulties with our own office building, we had to start over with a new office that we moved into soon after our business began to grow. The move was a difficult one, but we wanted to practice the same kind of medicine. God began speaking to me at that point. God said:

> I want you to practice the same kind of medicine you have always practiced except it's going to be a little different this time. I want you to establish a Christian clinic. From now on when you practice medicine, you are going to be ministering to patients. No longer are you just to address the physical and mental aspects of the men and women that I will send to you. You must address the spiritual aspect also. This is the plan I want you and your patients to follow.

God changed our practice totally, empowering us to discern spiritual things and to minister to our patients through the power of the Holy Spirit. When I started over with a new office and a new building, I also began to build my staff with Christian doctors, nurses and office personnel. Some astounding things began happening when we practiced medicine with prayer in the Holy Spirit. Incredible things happened in my life and through our clinic.

Practicing Medicine With God's Pathway to Healing

This book is the simple story of what God did in our medical practice in order to reveal His pathway of healing for our lives. Let me give you just a brief taste of what is to come in the following chapters.

Even though we are living in a great age of technology, I can unequivocally tell you that nothing or no one is more accurate in detecting disease than the Holy Spirit. I could share story after story with you about patients who came into the clinic and were touched by God.

One businessman came into the clinic for a colon exam. A colon exam can be painful, and when it becomes too uncomfortable we often terminate the exam. During every colon exam that I do, I pray and listen for God to give me specific directions. At a certain point in this man's exam I knew he was getting very uncomfortable. I was getting ready to end the exam when God clearly spoke to me, saying, "I want you to go on up higher in the colon."

I prayed, "Dear God, how can I put this man through any more misery?"

But God repeated, "I want you to go on up higher."

I moved the instrument up about two inches above the level where I had been ready to stop. As I did, I encountered a large growth which I believed was probably cancerous. As a result of that exam we were able to remove the cancer before it spread. It was removed from his colon without major surgery, and he was totally cured.

You see, God spoke. God speaks through the practice of medicine. A year later that same patient came in for a physical exam. Until that visit he did not know that I was praying over him when he was on the table for a colon exam a year earlier. This time we found some blockage in one of the arteries leading to his heart. Once again we had to pray for God's direction through another physical challenge.

God's pathway of healing can include the use of natural means of healing as well as supernatural healing. I had used natural, medical procedures to discover this man's artery blockage. But now I needed God's direction for the next step. I said, "God, what are we going to do? What is his pathway of healing?"

Prayer becomes the essence of a medical practice. At times God directs us to send a patient to the medical center. Sometimes the pathway of healing is a bypass, other times it's balloon angioplasty. In this man's case, although in the natural, medical wisdom would call for a bypass, but God spoke to me clearly, "This man is not to have a bypass."

I said, "God, what is Your pathway of healing for this gentleman?"

"His healing will come through prayer, nutrition, exercise and lifestyle changes," the Lord revealed to me. So I put him on nutrition and exercise programs. I retested his heart months later, and his EKG was normal. His blood flow had been restored without surgery. God had moved again.

God can move instantaneously and supernaturally when He chooses. One lady who came in for treatment had been to many different doctors because of pain in her shoulders. The cause of such pain is difficult at times to diagnose. Before I examined her I had prayed, seeking God. Her X-rays were normal, and nothing showed up during her examination. I said, "Ma'am, I don't know what to tell you."

That's all I said to her. She got up and left the office. The next day she phoned and said, "Dr. Cherry, on the way out the front door, that pain in my shoulder totally disappeared. I haven't had a touch of pain since." God healed spontaneously and miraculously. The supernatural is an important, incredible aspect of practicing medicine. God's pathway of healing constantly astounds me. He has created such enthusiasm in my life that each day I cannot wait to get to the clinic to see what He is going to do!

God sends some tough cases to us. One time a lady came in and said, "Dr. Cherry, I have been to six doctors." When I heard her say that, I knew right away that we were in for a tough case. It's a dead give away when patients have been to six doctors and still have the same problem.

She described some strange symptoms: sudden shoulder pain would hit her accompanied by hip and knee pain. Then her bones would give way, and she would collapse.

Her doctors had finally decided this woman was a psychiatric case because she returned to the emergency room week after week. As she sat in front of me in my office I prayed, "Dear God, what kind of story is this. I have never heard of anything like it." Suddenly God whispered the name of a rare disease in my ear.

I had not heard of this particular disease since medical school. I couldn't even spell its name! Couldn't even pronounce the name of the disease! I had never seen a patient with this disease before. But I said to the woman, "Ma'am, I think I know what your problem is. We are going to send you down to the medical center and have some special tests run on you."

I called the specialist in the medical center and said, "I'm sending you a lady with Ehlers-Danlos disease."

The doctor said, "Well, maybe it is, but I doubt it. That's a very rare disease. It probably isn't that."

He called me back after he examined my patient and said, "No, she doesn't have Ehlers-Danlos disease."

"Yes, I believe she does," I stated. Here I was, a doctor who had never seen a case of this disease, yet I was contradicting the diagnosis of a rheumatology specialist who had probably studied this disease all his life. But I insisted, "Ehlers-Danlos is what she has. Let's send her over to Baylor and call in a specialist, a geneticist!"

He said, "I think it's a waste of time, but if that's what you want, we will." He called the specialist.

Later I got a call from the geneticist, who said, "Dr. Cherry, we have a most unique case here of Ehlers-Danlos disease. I have never seen one quite like it." Upon further questioning of this patient, it turned out that most of the members of her family had had the same disease for as long as thirty years. Yet no doctor had ever diagnosed it accurately. They are still tracing back the history on that woman's family. That's the working of the Holy Spirit in a modern medical practice. He is the one who will "guide you into all truth" (John 16:13, NIV). Only God could have revealed that disease to me.

In this book, I will share stories of how God moves to heal in His pathway of healing. I share these stories to build your faith and, from the perspective of a medical doctor and teacher, to assure you from God's Word that there is a unique pathway for your healing. I want to encourage you to be willing to seek Him through both His natural and supernatural ways of healing.

I know what God has done in my life, and I know what God has done in the lives of my patients. He can do the same in your life! He is the Lord that healeth thee (Ex. 15:26). By His stripes you were healed (Is. 53:5).

God's Pathway of Healing

Two women came to me as patients with cancerous tumors. After numerous tests and prayer for God's leading, the first woman decided to have surgery to remove her malignant tumor. I felt, however, this might not be God's pathway of healing for her. Advising her to hold off the surgery, we set ourselves in agreement for her healing. I then suggested subsequent tests. Another X-ray was taken, and miraculously, there was no sign of the tumor. Further tests confirmed that God had supernaturally healed her without surgery.

A second woman with a malignant tumor went through extensive tests and intense prayer for her condition. She insisted that God would heal her supernaturally. Refusing any treatment in the natural, she angrily left my office because I would not agree with her that God would heal her in the way she desired and in her timing. God had actually shown me that her pathway to healing was through surgery. Her cancer was localized with no metastasis (spreading). I am convinced she could have been completely healed by the surgical procedure. Nonetheless, she wanted God to heal her supernaturally. She would not accept a natural course of medical treatment to achieve her healing. I still agonize over how simple the operation and healing would have been for her. Just a few months after she left my office she died from cancer. She had refused to walk in God's pathway of healing for her.

In the coming pages, I will share with you how God uses both natural and supernatural ways to heal. In the first part of this book, we will discover together:

- God's pathway of healing
- God's promises about healing and His healing covenant
- God's original health plan
- The power and authority God has given believers over disease
- Five spiritual principles of healing

In the second part of this book, we will uncover some specific natural ways that God has provided to prevent disease and to eliminate some of the destructive behaviors and eating habits that ravage our bodies.

Be assured that Linda and I are praying for you as you read this book. We are believing that through the Holy Spirit, God will reveal what your pathway of healing is for health, prosperity and abundant life in Christ Jesus.

Chapter 3

DOCTOR and the WORD

GOD HAS A PATHWAY
TO YOUR HEALING

An eighty-one-year-old lady came into the clinic for a complete, comprehensive examination. She wasn't experiencing any problems in her body; she just wanted to be certain she was in good health. She also wanted to know if there was anything else she needed to do in the natural to take care of her temple.

You might ask, "Why should a Christian who believes in divine health get a physical examination?" Paul said that we should not be unaware of the schemes or devices of the enemy (2 Cor. 2:11). This biblical concept has become a guiding principle in our clinic as we examine patients. Often the attacks of the enemy are very subtle. Our goal is to uncover the enemy's schemes at a very early stage.

One of Satan's most vicious attacks upon Christians is on their physical bodies, simply because the body is the temple that contains the indwelling Spirit of God. This elderly lady needed to hear the good news that I was able to give her after I finished her examination. She was in very good health. Just seeing God's hand of protection on her body gave "health to [her] body and nourishment to [her] bones" (Prov. 3:8, NIV).

Many older patients who come in for checkups have no intention of slowing down. Their attitude says, "I'm going to come in and get myself fine-tuned because I've got a lot left to do." We saw an elderly woman from the Southwest who was eighty years old. She had some annoying symptoms in her body and was somewhat confused about some of the medication she was taking. She had developed gout several months earlier and had been given a medication to take, which cleared the gout up in several weeks. However, she developed another attack of the disease. Finally she came to our clinic, seeking someone who would minister to her, pray and really seek the Holy Spirit for an answer to her problem. After I examined her, I said, "You know, I really feel led of God to put you on a different kind of medicine."

"Why is that?" she asked. "The other one worked even though it took awhile."

I said, "Well, the medicine that we are going to use for you will stop this pain — not in several weeks but much sooner."

She did not argue with me. She just said, "Let's get on with it, then." Along with the medication, we gave her a nutrition plan to avoid future attacks of gout.

We also had discovered that her blood pressure was high. She was already on a blood pressure medication but was not satisfied with it. She said, "This medicine doesn't make me feel right."

I said, "Well the reason is because you need to be on a different form of this medicine." So we changed her medicine. These were just little things to fine-tune her health. The gout was not going to kill her, but it would certainly slow her down and be very painful. So we gave her something to take for a day or two to clear up her symptoms — and it worked!

You might ask, "Dr. Cherry, why didn't you just cast the disease out and let her be healed supernaturally?" If the Holy Spirit had instructed me in that direction I would have. But there are different pathways for healing, and we need to look into each person's unique pathway.

The pathway of healing that God has for you now may be different from the one He has for someone else even though you may have similar health problems.

In the past I treated all my patients in the same manner. I did what I was taught to do in medical school. It did not matter how different their situations were or how God might be moving differently in their lives.

I realize that the Holy Spirit works differently in each individual, directing a pathway of healing for that particular person. We are each fearfully and wonderfully made.

It's wonderful to read in the Scriptures about the miraculous healings by Jesus. But sometimes we wonder if Hebrews 13:8 is true, "Jesus Christ is the same yesterday, today, and forever." These questions come to mind:

- Is Jesus really the same yesterday, today and forever?

- Are the same things happening today?

46

- Is there a difference in the way God heals today compared to healings in the Bible?

- What are the ways that healing is manifested today?

When Jesus was on earth, sophisticated medicine did not exist. No intricate technology was available. However, people were being healed supernaturally. They also received healing in other ways through a process or a pathway that led to their healings. For example, the ten lepers were healed "as they went." The blind man was healed as mud and saliva were applied to his eyes.

Healings take place today in the context of modern times, both through natural medicine and through the supernatural move of God's healing power through the Holy Spirit.

God's Pathway to Your Healing

God has a pathway that will lead to your healing. There are basic biblical truths and principles that underlie all healings. Understanding these scriptural truths and listening to the Holy Spirit will empower you to discover God's pathway to healing for you. I would like to share some of the basic scriptures which help us to find God's pathway.

Pathway of Healing Principles

1. God has a specific pathway just for you.

Luke 17 illustrates one way that God's pathway of healing works. Here is the story:

> Now it happened as He went to Jerusalem that He passed through the midst of Samaria and Galilee. Then as He entered a certain village, there met

Him ten men who were lepers, who stood afar off. And they lifted up their voices and said, "Jesus, Master, have mercy on us!" So when He saw them, He said to them, *"Go, show yourselves to the priests."* And so it was that *as they went,* they were cleansed. And one of them, when he saw that he was healed, returned, and with a loud voice glorified God, and fell down on his face at His feet, giving Him thanks. And he was a Samaritan. So Jesus answered and said, "Were there not ten cleansed? But where are the nine? Were there not any found who returned to give glory to God except this foreigner?" And He said to him, *"Arise, go your way.* Your faith has made you well" (Luke 17:11-19, italics added).

Notice the phrases I have italicized for you. The lepers were not healed immediately. They had to go and show themselves to the priests. There was a path they had to follow. As they went they were cleansed. The leper who returned was told by Jesus to "arise, go your way."

Recall the example of this principle that we mentioned earlier when Jesus healed a blind man (John 9:1-7). Again the healing was not immediate. Jesus used clay — a natural substance — to anoint the blind man's eyes. Furthermore, the man had to go his way and wash in order for the healing to be effective.

Many times the pathway to healing can be found only through a revelation of the Word of God. The Word can set you free and start you on a path that will lead to your healing. These two passages of Scripture describe the ways that Jesus gave specific instructions for healing. The lepers in Luke 17 and the blind man of John 9 had to follow a pathway and had to take specific action. Only then were they healed.

Another biblical illustration of this principle can be found in the story about Naaman (2 Kin. 5). An influential and powerful man, Naaman expected God to heal him instantly from his leprosy without any effort on his part. In those old covenant days God manifested Himself through prophets, priests and kings. In this case the leper sought Elisha, the man of God. Elisha did not come to meet him and heal him as Naaman thought he would. "Elisha sent a messenger to say to him, 'Go, wash yourself seven times in the Jordan, and your flesh will be restored and you will be cleansed'" (2 Kin. 5:10, NIV).

Naaman became angry about these instructions from Elisha and said, "I thought that he would surely come out to me and stand and call on the name of the Lord his God, wave his hand over the spot and cure me of my leprosy" (v. 11). Do you see? Naaman had expected God to heal him instantly in the way he wanted. Does this sound familiar in the church today? God had a specific pathway for Naaman's healing that was different from Naaman's expectations. So Naaman went away in a rage at the man of God and at God Himself.

Finally Naaman got over his anger, surrendered his expectations, decided to be obedient and "went down and dipped himself in the Jordan seven times, as the man of God had told him" (v. 14). At first, Naaman didn't want God's pathway of healing for himself. He finally surrendered to God's way and set aside his own expectations.

You may be feeling as Naaman felt. You may be angry with God and with other servants of the Lord — Christian doctors and pastors — because they have not responded in the way you expected. Do you want to hear from God and be healed, or do you want to keep going around the mountain of your illness?

2. Pray and seek God for your pathway of healing.

These stories confirm how important it is that we pray

about the pathway for our healing. We cannot list the many different ways that Jesus healed and simply choose one that suits us for our healing. Rather, we need to pray and seek God's specific plan. We have seen God open up many pathways for people to receive their healing as they pray and seek Him. Scripture even commands that we pray about our healing.

> Is anyone among you sick? Let him call for the elders of the church, and let them pray over him, anointing him with oil in the name of the Lord. And the prayer of faith will save the sick, and the Lord will raise him up. And if he has committed sins, he will be forgiven. Confess your trespasses to one another, and pray for one another, that you may be healed. The effective, fervent prayer of a righteous man avails much (James 5:14-16).

Instead of deciding what *we* want, we need to pray and ask God to reveal through the Holy Spirit what *He* wants. Prayer requires that we spend time alone with the Lord and the Word, waiting on the Holy Spirit. Jesus assured us that the Holy Spirit will guide us to all truth (John 16:13). Set aside your expectations and demands that God heal you in a certain way. Unless you can pray and hear from the Holy Spirit, it will be impossible for you to discover His pathway of healing for you.

3. God uses the natural and supernatural to heal.

Don't limit God to your expectations of how He will heal you. As a Christian physician, I see people make this mistake over and over again. Consider the different ways Jesus healed people of blindness in the Gospels. Jesus used the natural substances of clay, saliva and water to effect healing in one blind man (John 9:7). Another time, Jesus simply touched the eyes of two blind men, and they were instantly healed (Matt. 9:27-31). The blind man at Bethsaida came begging for Jesus to touch and heal him. Jesus spit on his eyes and put His hands on the blind man. Then Jesus asked him if he saw anything. The man could see men, but they looked like trees walking. "Then He put His hands on his eyes again and made him look up. And he was restored and saw everyone clearly" (Mark 8:25).

I want you to see that in all three instances Jesus used a different pathway of healing, using both natural and supernatural means to minister God's healing power. God uses doctors, medicines, herbs, nutrition, supplements, exercise, prayer and miraculous interventions of all kinds to heal us.

At times God's healing is spontaneous and instantaneous. Other times healing is a process and requires patience and perseverance as our healing is gradually manifested.

Don't misunderstand me. God can and does use doctors. But thank God there is a growing group of Spirit-filled doctors who believe in prayer and are not confined to just one way of healing. There are too many surgeries being performed. There is too much medication being prescribed. There are pathways that God has for His people that may deviate from standard, traditional medicine and treatment as we are taught in medical school. God's ways, though, are better than our ways.

Linda and I find some of the things that happen in our clinic to be quite interesting. Most people who come in are Christians and have their minds set on the thought, *I'm not going to have surgery.* However, by the time they leave God has moved on everybody, and we often discover God's pathway of healing is indeed surgery. Others come in insisting they don't want to continue on their medication. But God's Spirit moves, and by the time they leave they agree to continue taking it. Some patients who come to us are taking a lot of medicine. God often shows us that His pathway is to get off some, or all, of the medications.

Getting our minds locked on a certain way that we believe God has to move to heal us can be our biggest enemy. If we just let God move as He chooses, giving complete liberty to the Holy Spirit, His best for us will happen in our lives, and we will receive our healings.

God's ideal way is not medicine or surgery. It is to walk in divine health. However, often because of disobedience, rebellion and ignorance of His health laws, we must use medicine or have surgery. Thank God that He has a backup plan for us!

In every situation Linda and I always pray that no surgery or medicine will be necessary and that people will simply be healed and will walk in divine health. But we must be careful because too many Christians die an early death and that's sad. For example, on their own, without God's leading, they may choose to stop taking their medicines. That is very dangerous. They may say, "I have diabetes. But I'm never taking medicine or insulin again because I'm healed." Do not walk in fear. But if you believe you have been healed of diabetes, get a test. Work with your doctor. Don't be foolish. If you are healed supernaturally, God will confirm it. It is not a sign of faltering faith to confirm medically God's healing touch.

The key focus for our medical practice is being able to follow the Holy Spirit and find the pathway of healing for each person. I want to share some examples of how God's pathway of healing has worked.

God's Pathway of Healing at Work

Some patients come to us with mental problems such as depression and panic attacks. Many times their symptoms are similar. However, we have discovered that God has a different pathway of healing for each patient.

I have been studying a lot about the realm of mental illness lately. The reason why is because in many cases mental illnesses, insanity and so forth are the result of demonic influences. There are many examples of people who have been prayed for with the laying on of hands and subsequently, demonic spirits have been cast out in the name of Jesus. The individuals have been set free instantly. But not all mental illness is the result of a direct demonic influence. The specific source of a disorder may not be demonic but rather a physical imbalance.

Let me give you an example. Perhaps an individual has a stomach problem. The source of that problem is the enemy, Satan. Jesus warned that Satan is seeking to kill, steal and destroy (John 10:10). But the person's problem is not demon possession. He or she does not have demons in the stomach. The problem may be caused by a virus; or perhaps the person ate the wrong food; or the stomach may be producing too much acid; or the person may have a bacterial infection.

The same thing can happen in the mental realm. In other words, an actual physical problem may be causing a mental reaction. Often the problem is a chemical imbalance.

I had a patient tell me strange tales of things that were going on in her mind, peculiar thought patterns and the like. If she had gone to a secular doctor, he may well have institutionalized her. She was saying all kinds of bizarre things and using vulgar language. God told me to pray for the lady. That's all He told me. No medicine, nothing. God said, "You just pray and speak to those spirits, and she'll be free." And that's exactly what I did. That lady is now free.

On the other hand, another patient came in with another type of bizarre thinking. Through the Holy Spirit, God told me specifically that this person had a chemical imbalance and needed to be on medicine. Notice with one patient God used supernatural means to heal, and with the other He used medicine.

You may ask, "Why in the world does it work that way?" I don't know why it works that way. I don't know why Jesus used mud and saliva to heal the blind man. All I'm trying to do is listen to God for His plan.

We have seen mature, Christian church members that have developed chemical imbalances. Some well-meaning Christians think that all mental problems are caused by demonic manifestations. We treated a woman who was acting like the Gadarene demoniac (see Mark 5:1-20). Every time this poor lady turned around someone was casting a devil out of her. But nothing worked. This woman had a strong faith in Jesus Christ, but there were times when she would completely lose control of herself. She heard strange voices and constantly felt as if her hair was crawling with bugs, so she would wash it several times each day. She would also suffer from sudden anxiety attacks.

As I examined her and then prayed for God's direction in her treatment, God told me that she had a chemical imbalance. I put her on a medicine and within two weeks she was perfectly normal with no trace of a mental problem.

As Spirit-filled Christian doctors and patients we must know and apply the Word, using both supernatural and natural means as His Spirit directs. We do not want to miss God's healing pathway, instead we want to experience the fullness of God's healing for our lives.

My "Little Red Book"

We've talked about the Scriptures. The Word of God is

unchanged. Jesus is the same today as He was yesterday. The power of God to heal is unchanged. But we need to see the manifestations of healing. I'm going to share some stories from my "little red book." This book is one in which I enter a record of each healing we see at our clinic in Houston. We see patients come from all over the world with all kinds of problems. They come here frustrated and suffering, and God moves on their behalf as we pray together. They are able to find the solution to their problems through the Holy Spirit. Periodically Linda and I like to go to this little book and share the stories about the miracles and healings that have actually taken place.

One incredible story happened some time ago concerning a forty-one-year-old lady that came into our clinic. This lady had been to eight different doctors. I have no idea what her medical expenses were, but she had really suffered at the hands of many doctors. I could not believe it when she began to unfold her medical history. For years she had been suffering from chest pain. She complained of irregular heartbeats. She had been to two different cardiologists who had argued and disagreed over what was wrong with her. One said it was mitral valve prolapse but the other doctor disagreed.

She also described muscle aches that affected her whole body. Cramping occurred in her legs. She had pain in her esophagus and chest area when she swallowed. She complained of temperature elevations, nausea, faintness and dizziness. She had been given nerve conduction tests which inserted small needles into the skin. She had been given an echocardiogram, a CAT scan and two upper GI series. She was checked for lupus. In all, eight specialists had been unable to find out what was wrong with her, so she came to our clinic. She knew that the Holy Spirit was in our office. She knew that God alone had the answer to her illness. Together with me she was seeking God's solution.

I listened to all of her symptoms. I knew she had been to some of the most highly trained specialists available. Imagine her situation. I prayed as she sought God for His pathway of healing for her.

Usually when I see a patient who has been to so many doctors I know that God is getting ready to move. The stage is set for the miraculous to happen. So I conducted an exam, talked to her, probed the situation with her and ran several tests. I checked every organ in her body, but I couldn't find a natural solution. So I simply prayed, "God, show me through the direction and leading of the Holy Spirit what's going on here." I have never seen such a variety of symptoms in a person her age for which there was no explanation. There was no disease in the medical textbooks that fit the pattern of symptoms she had.

As I prayed, her solution suddenly unfolded. I started asking her about her stress levels. Specifically, we began discussing her marriage situation. I had to probe to find out what the problem was. She appeared to be happily married, but as we talked tears ran down her cheeks. The Holy Spirit took over and enabled her to open up.

She said, "You know, Dr. Cherry, for years and years I've never trusted my husband. Years ago we were at an athletic event, and I saw him flirting with all of the women. I began to hear rumors that he was unfaithful to me." The tears poured down her cheeks. The truth was revealed that for years she had been carrying an emotional burden within of an unfaithful husband. She had never been able to deal with it. Without the Holy Spirit's intervention, no doctor or medical treatment could have ever healed her. But now she recognized that her pathway of healing her physical body began as she was able to heal emotionally through forgiving her husband.

Over a period of a few weeks her symptoms gradually began to disappear, and she eventually became totally free of all of them. This case demonstrates that in the midst of such modern technology, unless we have the Holy Spirit, our Comforter, the One the Bible says will lead us into all truth, we can suffer endlessly. Medicine focuses on the complaint instead of the source of the problem. Medicine had no answer for her kind of pain but the Holy Spirit did.

Doctors can't measure the emotional hurt that you feel inside your body. We can't measure the rejection and the pain you may be suffering. Sometimes the hurt is so intense it is suppressed beyond our conscious awareness. Yet the Bible clearly tells us, "As the bird by wandering, as the swallow by flying, so the curse causeless shall not come" (Prov. 26:2, KJV). Each and every illness (which is a curse) has a cause. In every patient experiencing baffling symptoms I realize there is an explanation and a reason. Jesus will lead us into all truth. Led by His Spirit, we can discover the cause of the problem.

A man came into our clinic with a back problem he had had for more than forty years. He had received the best counsel, best medical advice he could receive from a long-established, nationally renowned clinic. Still he had no relief from his hurting back. His Christian wife encouraged him to come to us. She had seen *The Doctor and the Word* on television and said to her husband, "I want you to go see Dr. Cherry. He is a Christian man." That I was Christian meant nothing to him. But he had heard about our clinic and wanted a complete checkup.

This man told me his whole story, relating what each qualified specialist had done for him. But he still hurt terribly. So I prayed, and the Holy Spirit revealed to me that he needed a certain medication. I prescribed that medicine, but he wasn't too enthusiastic about taking another pill. He had been on dozens. But reluctantly he took it. He called me back the next day and said, "Dr. Cherry, I don't know what it is, but two hours after I took that medicine I was totally free of pain for the first time in forty years."

Now that only can be the Holy Spirit. In no way am I bragging on me. It's just that I pray when I don't have enough sense to know what to do! There are 150 different medicines to use for back problems. How would I be able to know which one would work for him? I couldn't know, but I'm led as I ask the guidance of the Holy Spirit. I seek to be led; then the Holy Spirit opens the door. The Comforter has come to a medical practice. Praise be to God!

Throughout this book, I will share other cases from my little red book. In many different ways God has miraculously healed so many people who have come through the clinic. These words are being written to encourage you. There is a way out for you, your loved ones and your family. Seek His pathway through the Scriptures and prayer. Seek a Spirit-filled doctor and surrender your expectations for healing to God's plan for your healing. Remember these important principles:

- God has a specific pathway for your healing.
- Pray and seek God for that pathway.
- God uses the natural and supernatural to heal

Steps Toward God's Pathway of Healing

To begin God's pathway of healing for you, take the following steps:

1. Consult a Spirit-filled doctor if you can.

2. Know God's Word about healing. Memorize and know the healing scriptures at the end of this book. These primary scriptures must enter into your spirit daily.

3. Seek God, and pray, asking for the Holy Spirit to reveal His pathway of healing for you through any natural or supernatural means He chooses to use.

4. Do what He tells you to do. Listen to His voice. Work closely with your doctor if that is part of your pathway. Remember, there is wisdom in a multitude of counsel. Exercise your faith in God's power to heal you.

5. Receive the support and prayers of other Christians who will encourage you and minister to you in your time of need as they exercise with you the mighty prayer of agreement.

Now that we have established that God has specific pathways of healings for individuals, read on to discover how to pray with authority for your healing.

Chapter 4

DOCTOR and the WORD

GOD'S HEALING COVENANT

I am a medical doctor in the private practice of preventive medicine. I would like to share perspectives about God's way of healing from the vantage point of a physician. Healing is vital to all of us. It's essential that we understand God's healing covenant because disease is one of humanity's greatest enemies. Eventually all of us will face the ravages of diseases that attack our bodies or the bodies of our family members and friends. We need to understand how God wants us to function in this area of healing. In this chapter I'm going to share about a unique combination of a medical approach to healing and that of a spiritual approach. Perhaps you may not have heard healing taught in exactly the way I will share with you, but I think you'll find it fascinating, inspiring and filled with life for you and for those you love.

God's Healing Covenant

Disease came on the scene very quickly after the fall. After the fall of Adam and Eve, God came to walk with them in the cool of the day.

> But the Lord God called to the man, "Where are you?" He [Adam] answered, "I heard you in the garden, and I was afraid because I was naked; so I hid" (Gen. 3:9-10, NIV).

The first mention of disease in the Bible is the identification of Adam's fear. Fear was the very first evidence of disease that attacked the human race. Thus disease attacked man at the beginning of the Old Testament, and Jesus attacked disease at the beginning of the New Testament.

Jesus dealt with disease throughout the majority of His ministry. In His first sermon, after He was baptized and tempted in the wilderness, Jesus attacked the very basis of disease when He proclaimed:

> The Spirit of the Lord is upon Me,
> Because He has anointed Me
> To preach the gospel to the poor;
> He has sent me to heal the brokenhearted,
> To proclaim liberty to the captives
> *And recovery of sight to the blind,*
> To set at liberty those who are oppressed;
> To proclaim the acceptable year of the Lord (Luke
> 4:18-19, italics added).

Notice that healing is one of the five points in His first

sermon — "And recovery of sight to the blind." When Jesus healed, He always used a pattern to effect the healing. Matthew 4:23 describes one of the basic patterns that Jesus used as He healed.

> And Jesus went about all Galilee, teaching in their synagogues, preaching the gospel of the kingdom, and healing all kinds of sickness and all kinds of disease among the people.

The Word of God precedes His Healing.

The Word of God came first; then healing followed. Psalm 107:20 declares, "He sent His word and healed them, and delivered them from their destructions." I want to share with you how God's covenant in His Word promises healing to you and me. When His Word comes to you, healing will follow. We must know God's Word before we can discern the pattern of healing He wills to use in our lives. Let's explore God's Word together.

Healing under the old covenant

Jesus taught and practiced healing in the context of the old covenant. As a prophet, Jesus stands at the crossroad of the Old and New Testaments, ushering in the new covenant. In other words, He kept the law. Jesus asserted, "Do not think that I came to destroy the Law or the Prophets. I did not come to destroy but to fulfill" (Matt. 5:17). Jesus healed in such a way that God's covenant and promises were completely and totally fulfilled.

For example, a rich young ruler came to Jesus one day and said, "Good Teacher, what good thing shall I do that I may have eternal life?" (Matt. 19:16). Jesus said to him, "Why do you call Me good? No one is good but One, that is, God. But if you want to enter into life, keep the commandments" (Matt. 19:17, NIV).

Today if someone were to ask us how to have eternal life, we would say, "Believe in the Lord Jesus Christ." But Jesus was functioning under the old covenant.

This is extremely important: All the healings that Jesus performed under that old covenant were effected on the basis of what He was going to do on Calvary. This is a fascinating point and one we must understand. All the healings that took place under the old covenant were types and shadows of what was going to happen when Jesus died on Calvary. Jesus introduced a new beginning for mankind — the new covenant.

We see prophetic glimpses of the coming new covenant in Jesus Christ through the prophet Jeremiah.

> Behold the days are coming, says the Lord, when I will make a new covenant with the house of Israel and with the house of Judah — not according to the covenant that I made with their fathers...I will put My law in their minds, and write it on their hearts; and I will be their God, and they shall be My people (Jer. 31:31,33).

Jeremiah prophesied about the coming of a new covenant. Hebrews 8:6 verifies that covenant.

> But now He has obtained a more excellent ministry, inasmuch as He is also Mediator of a better covenant, which was established on better promises.

As Jesus healed He was looking ahead to the cross. The work that Jesus would accomplish at Calvary was the basis of all the healings that took place under the old covenant. Let's look at Scripture to see how Jesus developed His healing ministry.

Jesus' pattern for healing

Jesus had just finished giving the Sermon on the Mount when a leper came up to Him and said, "Lord, if You are willing, You can make me clean" (Matt. 8:1). Jesus not only touched and healed the leper, but He also made a fascinating statement to the leper.

> Then Jesus put out His hand and touched him, saying, "I am willing; be cleansed." Immediately his leprosy was cleansed. And Jesus said to him, "See that you tell no one; but go your way, show yourself to the priest, and offer the gift that Moses commanded, as a testimony to them" (Matt. 8:3-4).

Now, why in the world would Jesus make a statement like that? Why would He tell the leper not to speak to anyone and to go to a priest and perform the rituals under the old covenant?

To understand what Jesus was doing we must read a passage in Leviticus. To show this leper (and us) a pattern for healing, Jesus was referring to a law that God had given thirty centuries earlier.

> This shall be the law of the leper for the day of his cleansing: He shall be brought unto the priest. And the priest shall go out of the camp, and the priest shall examine him; and indeed, behold, if the leprosy is healed in the leper, then the priest shall command to take for him who is to be cleansed two living and clean birds, cedar wood, scarlet, and hyssop. And the priest shall command that one of the birds be killed in an earthen vessel over running water. As for the living bird, he shall take it, the cedar wood and the scarlet and the hyssop, and dip them and the living bird in the

blood of the bird that was killed over the running water. And he shall sprinkle it seven times on him who is to be cleansed from the leprosy, and shall pronounce him clean, and shall let the living bird loose in the open field (Lev. 14:3-7).

Do you see what Jesus was doing by sending the leper to the priest? Here is an example of supernatural healing. But in explanation of that healing, Jesus showed a perfect picture of the work of the cross. There was a bird, wasn't there? That bird had to be killed in what? In an earthen vessel. When Jesus became God in the flesh, Jesus was killed in an earthen vessel (His physical body), wasn't He? The blood of the bird — a type of Jesus — that was killed was sprinkled on the other bird which was set free (that's us!). Jesus was showing by example the fulfillment of a centuries-old pattern for healing. But at the same time He was pointing us to the time when He would establish a new covenant on the cross of Calvary when by His shed blood He would cleanse us from sin, heal us and set us free.

Jesus pointed out this same pattern for healing when He said:

And as Moses lifted up the serpent in the wilderness, even so must the Son of Man be lifted up (John 3:14).

I wondered why Jesus would take a person all the way back to the old covenant to show a picture of Himself, to show what He was going to do on the cross. The answer can be found in the twenty-first chapter of Numbers. The Israelites were once again in trouble. They had spoken against God and Moses, so the Lord sent fiery serpents that bit the Israelites causing many to die.

When the Israelites finally repented of their sin, Moses prayed to the Lord. God did a most peculiar thing: He didn't

65

remove the serpents. He didn't reach down from heaven and drive the serpents away from those people. That's what they expected. Rather, God told Moses, "Make a fiery serpent, and set it on a pole; and it shall be that everyone who is bitten, when he looks at it, shall live" (Num. 21:8).

Moses did exactly what God commanded. When the Israelites were bitten, if they looked upon the brazen serpent, they were healed. Why didn't God just remove the snakes? God wanted the Israelites who were living under the old covenant to have a prophetic picture of the way He would heal under the new covenant — through Jesus Christ who would crush the serpent and disease on the cross. When Jesus became sin for us on the cross, He crushed Satan and all his serpents of disease as Jesus took on Himself the sins of the world.

In John 3 Jesus was giving us a dramatic example of the pattern of supernatural healing. Jesus was preparing the way for that better covenant with better promises.

This pattern is exactly how we are healed. Just as the Israelites looked forward to the cross, in the same way we look backward to the cross for our healing. God is saying, "You have to look upon the remedy I've given to you for your healing."

Isn't it interesting that the symbol used today to identify the medical field of medicine is the caduceus — snakes on a pole? When a physician graduates from medical school, he or she will have this symbol from the Old Testament on a diploma or school ring. It testifies to the truth that Jesus crushed the serpent and disease on the cross and became our Healer and Physician. Every doctor — Christian or not — uses this symbol that lifts up Jesus as the source of all healing.

For the Israelites, what was the remedy? It was the serpent upon that pole. Under the new covenant, we look to the Lord Jesus Christ. We don't look to a serpent on a pole.

The Israelites, who looked to Moses for everything, were told not to look to Moses for their healing. God was saying, "No, you are not to look up to Moses. You are to look to that remedy upon that pole." God was prophetically revealing the coming Messiah, Jesus, to His people.

What does that means to us today? You are not to look to your doctor for healing. You are not to look to your pastor for healing. For your healing, you are to look to Jesus who was lifted up on the cross.

Jesus is saying to us, "Simply look at the cure. Don't dwell on your symptoms. Don't dwell on how bad things are." Whoever looked upon that pole in the Old Testament was healed. That's for us today. Everyone who looks upon Jesus who died for us on the cross can be healed today. It's for everyone, but we have to believe. Each individual Israelite had to look upon the remedy for himself. "And it shall be that everyone who is bitten, when he looks at it, shall live" (Num. 21:8). Faith must be exercised by each individual.

You can't always get healed in a prayer line, even though the prayer of agreement is powerful. Yes, the Bible tells us to pray one for another. But it's the individual who must claim and receive healing.

The serpent being lifted up in the wilderness was a tremendous example that God gave us of the old covenant pattern for supernatural healing. Today, the best news of all is that we have a better covenant with better promises — Jesus Christ heals through His shed blood on the cross.

Does God Only Heal Supernaturally?

Now I'm getting ready to shock you. Many of you are familiar with God's covenant with us for supernatural healing. But did you know that God's original ideal plan for healing was not in the realm of the supernatural?

Let me show you what I mean. Consider this: God's

original plan was that man would never get sick in the first place. This was His plan long before He introduced these supernatural means for people to get healed.

I want to show you a fascinating thing in the fifteenth chapter of Exodus. God introduced the Israelites to a concept they were not familiar with — healing!

> If you diligently heed the voice of the Lord your God and do what is right in His sight, give ear to His commandments and keep all His statutes, I will put none of the diseases on you which I have brought [or allowed] on the Egyptians. For I am the Lord who heals you (Ex. 15:26).

This is the first time God entered into His healing covenant with man. Do you know what's even more fascinating? Immediately after God introduced Himself as the Healer in Exodus, He started giving commandments about what the Israelites were to eat. The very next words that God spoke to Moses were, "Behold, I will rain bread from heaven for you" (Ex. 16:4). In other words, God reveals Himself as a healing God and then immediately gives instructions about what His people will eat. If God is always going to heal supernaturally, why would He be concerned with what the Israelites ate?

I want to show you another interesting scripture.

> So you shall serve the Lord your God, and He will bless your bread and your water. And I will take sickness away from the midst of you (Ex. 23:25).

The amazing fact of this text is that God was speaking to a group of people who had no sickness at all. Did you know that? Psalm 105:37 reveals that "He also brought them out with silver and gold, and there was none feeble [or sick] among His tribes." Not one Israelite was sick, yet God chose that time to enter into a healing covenant. Do you know what God is showing us?

---

*God is showing us that His perfect will
for our healing is that
we never become ill in the first place.*

Isn't that an amazing facet of God's will for us? I was amazed when I realized how God had positioned these Scriptures revealing His perfect way of healing for mankind. This is an important principle of healing.

After we do what we can do in the natural, God will act in the supernatural to provide for our healing. We must keep in mind that there are both natural and supernatural means of healing incorporated into God's healing covenant. We need to understand when and how God moves in the natural and when and how He moves in the supernatural to heal.

Jesus Used Both the Natural and Supernatural to Heal!

Jesus illustrated this very well in John 11. He demonstrated that there is a natural action we take and a supernatural remedy that He will perform. John 11 is the familiar story about Lazarus, who was dying. Those attending to the sick man sent word to Jesus, hoping that Jesus would come to Bethany and heal him. But Jesus delayed. Lazarus died four days before Jesus arrived.

Mary, Martha and the mourners had no idea what Jesus would do. Lazarus's sisters, Mary and Martha, did all they could do. They cared for Lazarus in the natural, and they contacted Jesus. They had seen the tremendous healings and miracles that Jesus had performed. Though they trusted God for a supernatural remedy, their brother died.

I would love to have been there to see their reactions to

Jesus. The suspense! Those who were standing around the tomb had to be thinking, *What will Jesus do?* Jesus walked up to the tomb and asked where Lazarus had been buried. Then the first thing that Jesus did was to look around and command, "Take away the stone" (v. 38).

Lazarus's mourners must have been baffled. Why in the world would this miracle-worker have to ask them to move a stone away? With a word Jesus could have moved the stone just as He had calmed the sea and stilled the storm (Mark 4:35-41). Why didn't Jesus just move the stone supernaturally? He had the power to do so! But it was because God always asks us to do what we can do in the natural before He acts supernaturally.

By asking the men to move away the stone, Jesus was setting forth a pattern. By example, Jesus was saying to those people, "If you will do the things that you can do — in other words, you roll away that stone — I'll raise the dead. I'll do the supernatural." Here's the pattern:

- Hear and obey God's Word.

- Look upon Jesus for healing.

- Take God-guided actions in the natural — do all you can do.

- After doing all you can do in the natural, look to God for supernatural healing.

This is the very same pattern that we saw in Exodus when God said, "Look at the serpent." When they heard, acted and obeyed in the natural, doing what they could do, God healed supernaturally.

Jesus still says, "You do what you can do, then I'll do the supernatural: I'll raise the dead." We are to do in the natural what we can. God uses both the natural and the supernatural to bring about healing.

Chapter 5

DOCTOR
and
the WORD

GOD'S ORIGINAL HEALTH AND NUTRITION LAWS

Y our pathway of healing may involve doing something natural such as using a natural, common substance. Or you may experience God's healing supernaturally. God alone will show you your pathway to healing. God gave us many health laws under the old covenant as mechanisms to protect our health. Some of the old covenant laws do not apply today. For example, the ceremonial laws — pictures, types and shadows that God used over and over again such as the sacrifices and the grain offerings — are no longer observed. They pointed to and were fulfilled in Christ and were done away with in the new covenant.

But there are other commandments in the Law that didn't disappear such as the Ten Commandments — the moral laws. We still honor our parents, love God completely, abstain from idolatry, murder, adultery, coveting and lying.

Many people get confused about the laws. We aren't law-keepers. We are not bound by that Law anymore.

> For Christ is the end [completion or fulfillment] of the law for righteousness to everyone who believes (Rom. 10:4).

In other words, our righteousness, our right standing before God is no longer dependent upon our obedience to the Law. We don't have to keep the Law any longer to be righteous. We are saved by grace through faith (Eph. 2:8-9).

However, Christ's fulfilling the Law did not change God's health laws. The health laws in the old covenant did not disappear. Those health laws were instituted as a means of protection for us, just like the Ten Commandments. We do not follow them out of ritual or obligation or because they impute any kind of holiness or righteousness to us. Rather, we follow God's health laws to protect our bodies, our temples, from sickness and disease. God gave us His healing covenant as a provision for our protection and blessing as we live for Him.

We must maintain a balance on this issue. We must be cautious about these laws. It is so easy for the church world today to become fragmented on the issue of healing. Some denominational factions believe all healing takes place in the natural sense — through doctors, medicines and hospitals. Other factions of Christianity say, "No, I don't have to follow any laws (health laws included) anymore. I just look to the supernatural Healer — to God." We need to maintain a proper perspective. God wants us to protect ourselves by observing natural health rules. He also wants us to seek His supernatural intervention in our lives when we need it.

There are many terrible diseases that tend to affect people, particularly in the United States. Heart disease and hardening of the arteries kill about 52 percent of all Americans. Cancer is the number two cause of death.

However, certain groups of people in this world are essentially free of hardening of the arteries, various kinds of heart disease and cancer. They have almost none of these diseases. The question that must be answered is, What are these people doing? These people may not know it, but they are following God's original health laws.

Isn't that fascinating? Whether people are saved or unsaved, when they knowingly or unknowingly line up with the Word of God, healing is at work in their bodies. Most of the people in countries relatively free of heart disease and cancer are following a diet that was introduced by God for their protection from the very beginning. It is His original plan for man's nutritional intake that protects the body.

God's Original Health Plan

God apparently thought this was so important to man that He did not allow the first chapter of the Bible to go by without introducing the health plan for man. From the beginning of creation, God developed a health plan to show humanity the exact way to live.

In Genesis 1:29, God first mentions what we should eat and put into our bodies, saying:

> Behold, I have given you every herb bearing seed, which is upon the face of all the earth, and every tree, in the which is the fruit of a tree yielding seed; to you it shall be for meat (KJV).

This particular scripture was given to man under ideal environmental conditions. It is actually a type of vegetarian diet which is based on fruits, vegetables and seeds. We can no longer survive easily on that type of diet. In fact, God Himself modified that nutrition plan later on in the ninth chapter of Genesis. Between the first and ninth chapters of Genesis, man rebelled against God by sinning. Humanity fell. There was also a great flood. A great judgment came on the face of the earth, and it affected everything upon the earth. Sin had infected creation. God's judgment of sin affected the soil, the plants, what we eat and how we live.

In the ninth chapter of Genesis, God made some changes in our nutrition because of man's rebellion. God said:

> Every moving thing that liveth shall be meat for you; even as the green herb have I given you all things. But flesh with the life thereof, which is the blood thereof, shall ye not eat (Gen. 9:3-4, KJV).

God was now adding some meat (flesh) into the diet. Some people still try to sustain their nutrition on a total vegetarian diet. That is difficult to do. Certain deficiencies such as in vitamin B_{12} and iron can occur without some meat (fish or chicken) in our diets. We need some meat — complete protein products — in our diets.

That doesn't mean that every moving thing should be part of our diets. God, through the Levitical dietary codes, told us specific types of food and meat in particular to eat and not to eat. I want to introduce you to the subject of nutrition as God instructed for our health.

Why Is God's Plan of Nutrition so Important?

As a medical doctor, I practice preventive and diagnostic medicine. In our Houston clinic, our whole thrust is to keep people healthy. Perhaps the most critical area in my treatment of patients is in the area of nutrition.

You may ask, "How can nutrition be so important?" Well when we begin looking at the statistics, we find a very interesting pattern. Six out of the ten leading causes of death in this country are directly related to what we eat. It is estimated by some that 50 to 60 percent of cancer may relate to our food intake. The matter of what we put into our mouths is critical (see Ex. 16).

God did not give us dietary laws to put us into bondage, but rather it is to protect us.

Our right standing with God is not connected to our observance of biblical health codes. However, God's ideal pattern for us is to stay healthy and learn how He designed us to operate. We need to discover how God wants us to function in nutrition because it is part of our obedience to God's pathway of healing.

God provided a detailed plan of nutrition for His people. He provided manna to the Israelites (Ex. 16), describing it as being like coriander seed (Ex. 16:31). He told the people to gather it in the morning and eat it. In the evening they were to eat quail (Ex. 16:12-13), thereby God added meat into their diets.

God was specific with the Israelites about eating. I want to be specific with you about nutrition, introducing you to God's health plan now. I will go into more depth in the second half of this book.

We must understand these concepts. The Bible was not written as a nutrition manual, but it was written to give us a pattern for abundant and healthy living. Jesus came not only to give us life but to give us a more abundant life (John 10:10). To have that abundant life, we must apply the lasting truths revealed in Scripture about nutrition.

What Can I Eat in God's Health Plan?

"Well, Dr. Cherry," you say, "how should I eat? What

should I buy from the store? What should I avoid eating, and what foods should I eat? What is included in God's plan?" Let's take a closer look at God's health plan. As we look, we will discuss several myths about nutrition which hinder us from following God's health plan for our bodies.

Myth #1: Protein is the perfect food.

What protein should I eat? There is a great myth in this country regarding protein. As a result, the enemy has deceived us in this area.

Many of us were raised with the idea that protein was a perfect food, the ideal food to eat. Did you know that protein is one of the most difficult substances for the human body to digest? Only about 10 percent of our dietary intake should be in the form of protein. After Noah and the flood, protein was added to our diets by God in the form of meats, fish and quail. We do need protein in our diets, and we need some of our protein through meat — fish and chicken — and the rest from vegetables.

In our clinic, we try to get our patients to make a shift to eating more fish and chicken instead of red meat. Fish and chicken are high protein sources with low fat levels that we will discuss later in the book.

Myth #2: We need protein supplements.

When you start thinking about your body — the temple of the Holy Spirit — and how to take care of it nutritionally, don't jump on the wagon that says, "Well, I need to go on protein supplements." That's the last thing you need to do. It's a myth. We need to keep our protein intake constant at about 10 percent of our total diet. You say, "Well, Dr. Cherry, if I'm not going to eat protein, where am I going to get most of my calories? Where am I going to get most of the substance in my diet?"

Myth #3: Meat is our primary source of calories and energy.

Many people believe that meat or protein should be the primary source of our calories for energy. This is another myth.

Actually, the primary source in our diet for energy should be carbohydrates. God referred to this when He indicated that manna was "bread from heaven." He was describing the eating of complex carbohydrates!

Ways to Eat Right!

The people in cultures today who eat foods high in complex carbohydrates are essentially free from heart disease and strokes. Often their diets contain as much as 80 percent carbohydrates. That's a fascinating concept because it's the same pattern of food intake that God gave us under the old covenant laws. You may be thinking, *But I cannot go out and buy manna. And I don't even know what coriander seeds are.* Let me share with you what you can do.

There are the four nutritional groups which should make up the substance of your dietary intake. These groups comprise what we today call the complex carbohydrates.

1. Green and yellow vegetables

You should have three or more servings of green and yellow vegetables each day. People who eat these foods as part of their cultural diets are essentially free of the diseases that kill so many of us in this country.

There are four particular groups of vegetables that we focus in on in this area of carbohydrates that have been shown consistently to offer high protective effects from cancer. This fact is verified in medical journal after medical journal. To remember these four vegetable groups, think of two *B*s and two *C*s. The two *B*s are broccoli and brussels sprouts. The two *C*s are cabbage and cauliflower. Maybe those are the same things your mother told you to eat years ago. Yes, Mama was right, wasn't she? Population groups with high consumption of those vegetables show a marked decrease in the incidence of many internal cancers. We're not sure what it is. Perhaps it's the chemicals such as beta carotene, luteins and indoles found in these foods that work to protect us.

2. Grains

Observe that God has given us many of these substances to protect ourselves. These include rice, potatoes, breads and cereals. We need two or more servings of grains each day.

3. Fruits

Eat at least three servings of fruit each day. Citrus fruits, cantaloupe, strawberries and apples are exceptionally good. There are many fruits that are very high in nutrient value and excellent for suppressing cancer cell development and lowering cholesterol.

4. Beans and peas

We only need three or four servings of beans and peas each week, simply because they are higher in caloric intake and can increase our weight.

5. Fiber

Where does fiber fit into our diet? You may have read a lot about fiber. Fiber intake in our diet is critical. We can get fiber from many sources — vegetables, fruits, cereals — but I tell all of our patients to be sure that they are getting enough fiber by adding a cereal to their nutritional intake.

It is preferable to eat cereal early in the morning. We recommend high fiber cereals to our patients, such as cereals with added bran. There are many sugar-coated cereal products available, and you need to be very careful of these. We have found what we consider a very scientific principle to help guide our patients to select the right kind of cereals: We tell them to get a cereal and taste it. The more it tastes like ground-up tree bark, the better it is for you! Some of these bran cereals are hard to get down. It was hard for me to find a cereal high in fiber that I could enjoy eating. Some that are available now have a tolerable taste. The bran gets us back to the concept God introduced of eating seeds.

Bran is actually the seed coat of seeds such as oats and wheat. This bran coating remains on the seed. God referred to such seed in Genesis 1:29. Bran has protective agents in it, and people who are on a high fiber intake have a lower incidence of colon cancer, our number one internal malignancy. Also their blood fat levels of cholesterol triglycerides tend to drop. Some recent studies have shown there may be a particular benefit to oat bran. Oat bran cereals are now available. People who eat one-third of a cup of bran per day have been shown to have significantly reduced blood fat levels of cholesterol and triglycerides.

People who lived under the old covenant were following dietary codes that included bran, or seeds, as a part of their diet. Many of the Jewish people whom Jesus healed while He was on earth were obedient Jews who still followed the dietary codes of the old covenant. Isn't that fascinating when you stop and think about it? God does have a pattern for us to follow in the natural in order to maintain good health. That pattern began in the old covenant.

How many more healings would we see if we began lining up with God's Word? You see, that's the natural part that man has to do. Eating the right food is an action we can take in the natural for protection from disease. The time may come in your life, or in your family members' lives, when there is a need for a supernatural healing beyond anything that you can do. But you will have already done all you can in the natural in preparation for God's finishing supernatural touch.

God's Healing Covenant Protects Us

Let me show you specifically how our Father, out of His great love and mercy, desires to protect us from the ravages of disease. The devil came to kill, steal and destroy, but Christ came to destroy the works of the devil (John 10:10; 1 John 3:8). God has given us natural foods and substances to protect our bodies.

Cancer, for example, is a fearful disease in which the body actually turns on itself and loses control of cell function in the body. Cells begin growing and outgrowing their blood supply. Eventually they can kill the organism. But even before humanity knew what cancer was, God gave us provisions in His dietary laws through His healing covenant to prevent cancer.

Let me give you just one example to bring you up-to-date. Medicine is always trying to catch up with the Word of God. When a great medical discovery is made, we always find that the footsteps of God have preceded our own. Doctors, nurses, healing pastors and evangelists do not heal anybody — we simply offer treatment. It is God who brings our healing through the blood of His Son on Calvary.

In an article published some time ago in *The Journal of the American Medical Association (JAMA)*, researchers confirmed that seeds hold cancer at bay. The article stated that the incidents of major cancers, such as prostate cancer, breast cancer and colon cancer (those are some of our biggest cancer risks in this country) are significantly lower in populations whose diet is rich in seed foods such as maize, beans and rice. Some of the research is now pointing to the fact that there may be certain enzymes common to all seeds that will suppress the development of cancer cells.

I practice medicine in Houston, Texas, where a world renowned research center that does cancer research is located. A study was done at this hospital that determined that the protein from certain vegetable sources in seeds would inhibit tumor formation. The conclusion of this article in reference to protecting us from cancer states that a prudent diet would be one in which one-third to one-half of all protein is derived from seeds. Does this sound familiar? It should. Our Father said it thirty-five centuries ago at the beginning of creation!

Remember the principle for healing that we learned in this chapter: God has given us both the natural and supernatural for our pathway of healing. Study this book carefully, and do all that you can do in the natural to prevent disease.

God's healing covenant has been given to us so that we can know what to do in the natural in order to walk in health. However, there will be times when we need to cry out to God, praying for a supernatural healing. In the next chapter we will discover the authority and power we have in Christ Jesus to do just that.

DOCTOR and the WORD

POWER AND AUTHORITY OVER DISEASE

Good news! Through the blood of Jesus Christ we have power and authority over disease. First Peter 2:24 declares that we have been healed through the stripes of Jesus Christ. But how do we exercise the power and authority of our position in Christ?

One scripture lays the foundation for our authority.

> And God said, "Let us make man in our image, after our likeness: and let them have dominion over the fish of the sea, and over the fowl of the air, and over the cattle, and over all the earth, and over every creeping thing that creepeth upon the earth" (Gen. 1:26, KJV).

The key to our authority is, "Let them have dominion." You see, God created and designed man to have dominion on this earth. In that particular scripture we can envision the transfer of authority to man for all that God intended to do on earth.

God chose to function on earth through a man in the flesh because God had given man dominion over the earth. Understanding that perspective, we begin to see that the whole purpose for God's will was to act through us. That is why He desires that the temples through which He acts and moves — our bodies — are walking in divine health. God chooses to manifest Himself through human beings. He began with Adam. However, Adam chose to give up his dominion, surrendering his power and authority to the prince of the air, thus giving Satan a temporary lease over the earth until Jesus returns!

Because of the great rebellion of man on earth just before the flood, God again had to look for a man. Again God chose to act on earth through the natural body. He found and used a man — Noah — to effect His purposes for humanity.

God put within each one of us an intense desire to take care of our human bodies so that He might act through us for His glory. Every cell in your body strives for life. Every breath you take is for life. Our whole purpose on earth is to perpetuate life. We are to live life according to His purpose and will.

After generations of wickedness of man on earth spanning from Adam to Lamech (Gen. 5), God chose to act through a righteous man, Noah. The Bible says that Noah was the only human being who was righteous in the eyes of the Lord. God acted through Noah and his family to preserve the human race by means of the ark.

Later God looked to Abraham through whom God birthed the Hebrew race, out of which came ultimate life —

Jesus Christ. In Christ, the Word of God became a body and dwelt on the earth to fulfill God's perfect plan for life. Through the Son of man, God gave us the power and authority to exercise dominion over the earth. We are to take care of our bodies, for Jesus came to dwell in, redeem and heal them through the cross. As Paul writes:

> Do you not know that you are the temple of God and that the Spirit of God dwells in you? If anyone defiles the temple of God, God will destroy him. For the temple of God is holy, which temple you are (1 Cor. 3:16-17).

How Does God Give Us Authority Over Sickness?

Any time disease enters our bodies, our authority and ability to exert dominion on this earth are diminished in direct proportion to the disease's entrance into our bodies. Let's take a look at the things that God used in order to effect His purpose on earth to give us authority, power and dominion over sickness.

1. He has to have a body.

Thus when Jesus was conceived by the Holy Spirit, He fulfilled God's requirement to accomplish His plan through a body. That's one reason Jesus is referred to so often as the Son of man. The Word became flesh (John 1) and indwelt a human body so that humanity through Christ might regain authority and power over sickness, sin and death.

2. The body God needs must be free from sin.

God could not use just any body. He required a human being who was free of sin consciousness. That's the reason Jesus was conceived by the Holy Spirit. God indwelt a human body that was free of sin. The sin consciousness that had been passed down through each generation since Adam was not present in Jesus because He was conceived supernaturally by the Holy Spirit. If God is to use us, our bodies must also be freed from sin consciousness. We must be cleansed of sin by the blood of Jesus Christ (1 John 1:9)

3. God requires a body that is indwelt by the Holy Spirit even as Christ was indwelt and empowered by the Spirit.

Now consider this: Jesus did nothing in ministry for thirty years. His ministry began when this third requirement had been met. The Holy Spirit descended upon and empowered His body to exercise God's authority and dominion on the earth. After Jesus' baptism, in the power of the Holy Spirit, He overcame Satan's temporary authority (Luke 4:1-13) and began His ministry in power. "Then Jesus returned in the power of the Spirit to Galilee" (Luke 4:14). Jesus was ultimately crucified and raised in body from the dead. Through Jesus' body, God defeated the dominion of Satan over the earth and destroyed the works of the devil — sin, disease and death (1 John 3:8)

We have physical bodies that God desires to use once they are indwelt by the Holy Spirit. We are to operate and flow in God's pattern of health on this earth. There are a lot of physical bodies on earth, and many of them are striving to be healthy. The world is making every effort to walk in health, from joining health spas to taking all kinds of vitamins and supplements to eating right. God built the desire to be healthy into the nature of man. We yearn to take dominion over our bodies and have power over the world around us. However, that desire can only be realized as we are born again by the Spirit of God and become the temple — body — of God. Just as Christ was born of the Spirit, we also need to be born of God's Spirit.

But as many as received Him [Christ], to them He gave the right to become children of God, to those who believe in His name: who were born, not of blood, nor of the will of the flesh, nor of the will of man, but of God (John 1:12-13)

Jesus answered, "Most assuredly, I say to you, unless one is born of water and the Spirit, he cannot enter the kingdom of God" (John 3:5)

The three main factors in our human bodies that give us dominion on this earth are: Being born again of the Holy Spirit; being cleansed by Jesus' blood and freed from sin consciousness; and being indwelt by the presence of the Holy Spirit.

We want to keep our bodies healthy so that we might honor and glorify God and be used by Him in our bodies. God's purpose for us is to give us, as His children, dominion, power and authority over the earth. As a born-again believer you have the authority in your body to exercise God's power over sin and sickness. Are you exercising your authority? God wants you to preserve and to take care of your body so that you might exercise dominion as a child of God over the earth

Can Our Thoughts and Words Take Authority Over Sickness?

We can understand exactly how God designed us to function. We can be in optimal health in our physical bodies and still need to take authority to exercise the God-given power for overcoming the evil that attacks and torments us. To be healed and to walk in health, we must recognize that the source of our authority is God — not our human thoughts and efforts. At the time of creation God gave man dominion and authority over the earth. After the fall, humanity deserted God but still tried to take dominion based on its own resources.

In Genesis 11:6 God observed:

> Behold, the people is one, and they have all one language; and this they begin to do: and now nothing will be restrained from them, which they have imagined to do (KJV).

Now this is a familiar story, but I want to paint a vivid picture for you. This is the story of the tower of Babel. As pagan unbelievers discussed how to build a tower to heaven, they said to one another:

> Go to, let us build us a city and a tower, whose top may reach unto heaven; and let us make us a name, lest we be scattered abroad upon the face of the whole earth (Gen. 11:4, KJV).

God heard their wicked plans to take illegitimate authority by attempting to be gods themselves. In that scripture God is showing us a key insight into the way He designed man to operate. These people were heathen, unsaved people who were seeking to grasp a power that God put in man — the ability to accomplish through imagination and unity anything they could conceive.

Think of the power revealed in that passage. In these unsaved people God saw a strong imagination — a strong image of a city and a tower whose top might reach to heaven. Because of that image, God came down to earth to look into this matter. He knew the gravity of this matter. These wicked men had a potent thing going for them. Because they had one language, they spoke in unity and the flow of words that came out of their mouths was powerfully authoritative. God decided quickly to make a change, and He confounded their language and confused their imaginations.

This is an essential key for understanding the power that God gave us to overcome disease. With the power of God at work in our lives believers can picture (have an image) wellness in our bodies and speak in unity, confessing what God's Word says about our healing. Believers have the authority in Christ to speak with power to disease and sickness.

At this point you may ask, "How do I deal with disease that is already in my body? I've been diagnosed with an incurable disease. The doctors give me no hope of recovery. Dr. Cherry, what do I do now?" For example, you may have a cancer in your body that has metastasized (spread throughout your entire body). Later in this book I will devote a chapter to cancer and its treatment through nutrition. Let me tell you I have patients who have been totally healed of cancer. Believers who have been supernaturally healed have stood in agreement and unity in order to focus their imaginations and thoughts upon the Word of God.

Our thoughts are powerful weapons against disease and sickness. We must get our thinking right — lined up with God's Word — in order to fight off and overcome disease.

Start by saturating your thoughts with God's love for you. Read 1 Corinthians 13; John 3 and 1 John 4. Take every thought captive (2 Cor. 10:5) and develop a feisty, fighting attitude to take the kingdom of this world with its sickness and disease by force (Matt. 11:12).

I want to point out an interesting thing from the first

chapter of Genesis. Eleven times God spoke or by His word called the created order into being. God uncovers something for us here. I invite you to do what I have done — underline all the verses in that chapter that refer to God speaking to His people. He is showing us the key to the way He designed us to function. We can see this same pattern in Mark 11:23. God exerted His authority on earth through His words. These words came out of the imagination, out of the mind of God Himself, and they manifested themselves through His Word.

Jesus applied this principle in Mark 11:23.

> For assuredly, I say to you, *whoever says* to this mountain, "Be removed and be cast into the sea," and does not doubt in his heart, but believes that those things *he says* will be done, he will have whatever *he says* (italics added).

Three times the believer speaks words in this verse. So God is showing us a pattern. Words are powerful. God introduced and created the world through His words. Jesus speaks a word and people are healed. He commands us to speak in faith and miracles happen. The Bible declares, "Death and life are in the power of the tongue, and those who love it will eat its fruit" (Prov. 18:21).

The words we believers speak have the power to overcome disease and destruction. Suppose you have a health problem in your physical body. How do you address this need? The Bible instructs us to keep His Word in front of our eyes (Prov. 4:20-21). If you are hurting and desperate in your body to be free from pain, disease and destruction, speak God's Word.

Frankly, for many of the diseases that we face such as cancer or AIDS, medical science has no answer. With certain diseases, we have reached the end of human ability. What do we do next? We may face a chronic problem of pain with an illness like arthritis. Medicine cannot cure this chronic disease, but God's Word gives us power and authority. Walking in divine health is available to every believer.

One scripture I frequently share with my patients is, "the curse causeless shall not come" (Prov. 26:2). Part of the curse which came after the fall was disease. Every curse has a cause. As Christians we have the authority and power to speak God's Word over the curse and its cause.

If you have an illness or disease, begin to think and speak three specific scriptures. Write these down. Mark them in your Bible. Hide them in your heart.

> He [Jesus] is despised and rejected by men; a man of sorrows, and acquainted with grief: and we hid as it were our faces from him; he was despised, and we esteemed him not.
>
> Surely he hath borne our griefs, and carried our sorrows: yet we did esteem him stricken, smitten of God, and afflicted. But he was wounded for our transgressions, he was bruised for our iniquities: the chastisement of our peace was upon him; and with his stripes we are healed (Is. 53:3-5, KJV).

> That it might be fulfilled which was spoken by Isaiah the prophet, saying: "He Himself took our infirmities and bore our sicknesses" (Matt. 8:17).

> Who Himself bore our sins in His own body on the tree, that we, having died to sins, might live for righteousness — by whose stripes you were healed (1 Pet. 2:24).

These passages reveal that part of our redemption through the shed blood of Jesus includes healing for our physical bodies. If you are hurting or have a medical problem, as a doctor my prescription would be:

- Read aloud these scriptures every day.

- Let the Word of God remain before your eyes.

- Speak the Word with your mouth.

- Take authority over sickness and disease in your body by seeing, reading, speaking and hearing God's Word.

Out of your spirit man where the Holy Spirit indwells can come forth God's Word to bring life to your physical body.

We are "partakers of the divine nature, having escaped the corruption that is in the world through lust" (2 Pet. 1:3-4). When you are born again into the family of God, your spirit man is recreated, becoming new and filled with life (2 Cor. 5:17). The Scripture reveals that our spirit man sustains us in our infirmities (Prov. 18:14). Your spirit man will sustain you through your illness as you feed on God's Word. The Word of God is the bread of life to your spirit man. Feed your spirit man the Word so that the divine nature within you can overcome the corruption in your flesh.

Let me show this to you in another passage.

> We know that whoever is born of God does not sin; but he who has been born of God keeps himself, and the wicked one does not touch him (1 John 5:18).

We know that anyone born of God does not knowingly or deliberately continue practicing sin. Christ carefully watches over and protects the believer. His divine nature within preserves us from the wicked one. The enemy cannot get a grip on the believer. This text declares that the devil cannot touch your spirit man. Now that's power and authority!

So get this into your imagination, into your mind as it is being renewed (Rom. 12:1-2). If the wicked men at the tower of Babel had power in their unrighteous imaginations, how much more power and authority does your born-again spirit man have when you imagine, think and speak God's Word!

Joel prophesied, "And it shall come to pass afterward that I will pour out My Spirit on all flesh" (Joel 2:28). Psalm 107:20 declares, "He sent his word and healed them, and delivered them from their destructions." As the Word of God goes forth from your spirit man into the world, you will see a revitalizing of life, a lengthening of your life, a fullness and an abundance of life.

We see the transforming power of God in the life of Jesus on the Mount of Transfiguration (Mark 9, Matt. 17). Christ's face shone white as the sun. Jesus didn't turn into God, but His human body was so transformed by God's Spirit that His whole countenance was changed. When Jesus descended from the mountain the people simply looked at Him with amazement (Mark 9:14). Why? Because the light and power of God was on Jesus. He radiated with power and life. That same life and power through the Holy Spirit lives within you. That's the divine nature of God in you.

> But if the Spirit of Him who raised Jesus from the dead dwells in you, He who raised Christ from the dead will also give life to your mortal bodies through His Spirit who dwells in you (Rom. 8:11).

Dwelling within you is the healing, life-giving Spirit of God. The Word goes forth, healing and delivering us from our destructions. There are some hindrances — like sin, bondage, rebellion and doubt — that block this divine flow from coming out of our spirit man and into our bodies. I want to ask you right now: Are you willing to trust God's power and authority dwelling in you through the Holy Spirit for your healing? Are you willing to act in faith to be healed?

Persistent in Faith, Believing for Your Healing

Faith is essential to healing.

Be persistent in your faith. As we will discover, the lack of faith is a major hindrance to healing. Faith is activated by our own words as they are spoken in agreement with God's Word (Mark 11:23-24). As you pray in faith, seeking God's healing power and authority in your life, remember to let go of past hurts, to forgive and to love others (Mark 11:25-26).

Know against whom you are fighting.

"For we do not wrestle against flesh and blood, but against principalities, against power, against the rulers of the darkness of this age, against spiritual hosts of wickedness in heavenly places" (Eph. 6:12). You must be persistent in prayer, persistent in speaking God's Word and persistent in believing on Christ. Don't give up. Give freedom to your spirit man to take authority and power in your life through the Holy Spirit to transform, heal and restore your body with the life of Jesus Christ.

Pray with power and authority.

How can you pray for supernatural healing with authority and power? Here is a summary of what I have been sharing with you in this chapter:

- Get God's Word into your spirit man, thoughts and words. We must get our thinking right to fight off disease. Start by saturating your mind with love which casts out fear and enables your faith to work. Learn to think on the right things (Phil. 4:8).

- Get the right attitude. You must have a feisty, fighting attitude toward disease in your body. "The violent take it [the kingdom of heaven] by force" (Matt. 11:12).

- Talk right. What you think and deposit into your spirit man from the Word of God must be spoken (Mark 11:23). Righteous and holy words must flow from your mouth like living water. Speak God's Word with authority, power and life. Declare the words of these verses aloud: Exodus 15:26; Isaiah 53:3-5; Matthew 8:17; and 1 Peter 2:24.

- Know the enemy, and persist in prayer (1 Thess. 5:17; Eph. 6:10-18), knowing that He who is in you is greater than the enemy whose works have been destroyed by Christ (1 John 3:8; 4:4).

Don't give up! In the following chapter we will look closely at five spiritual principles of healing.

Chapter 7

DOCTOR and the WORD

FIVE SPIRITUAL PRINCIPLES OF HEALING

In my medical practice there are certain specific spiritual principles that lead patients toward their healing in awesome ways. Through the leading of the Holy Spirit, God is directing us to review these principles with all of our patients who seek healing from specific problems. I want to share these principles with you. You may find yourself in a situation similar to the one in a letter I received from a patient in the Midwest. She writes:

> As a child of God, I know that Jesus carried my problems to the cross for me. I shouldn't have to learn to live with the twenty-four-hour pain the neurosurgeons have told me to expect. Dr. Cherry, I've been prayed for and prayed for, and I

fail to understand why I'm not receiving the fulfillment of my promise for divine healing. I would so
appreciate it if you and your wife would pray for
me. Possibly the Holy Spirit will reveal to you
what I'm missing.

This is just one example of the way people want God
to reveal the solution to their medical problems. Many
patients have said something like this to us at the clinic, "I
have this problem in my body. I have this pain in my body.
I've been prayed for and prayed for, and I can't understand
why I'm not receiving my healing."

One day a pastor came into our clinic who was seeing a
cardiologist in another city. He needed some answers as
well as guidance from the Holy Spirit about what to do for
his chest pain. We examined him, put him through tests
and prayed with him. God gave us a very clear diagnosis of
what his problem was — a blockage in an artery.

We developed a program to help reverse his problem. We
explained the steps that God showed us to this pastor, and
he had total peace about it. Near the end of the exam he
said, "Dr. Cherry, I'm a faith preacher. I've taught faith and
divine healing for years. To be honest with you, this is a little
frustrating to me. Here I am with a problem, having to do
certain medical things such as begin taking medication and
have medical tests. And frankly, it's a little difficult sometimes for me to explain my illness to my congregation."

The Five *P*s of Spiritual Healing

I want to go through a very concise list of steps that you
need to keep in your mind when you face a spiritual battle
similar to the ones this woman or this pastor were facing.
We are going to talk about five spiritual principles of healing. I like to refer to them as the five *P*s of spiritual healing.

1. Jesus is the Physician who heals.

Jesus is our healer. By His shed blood, we are healed. Disease never comes from God. It is part of the curse. Illness is often used as an attack of the enemy. Our own destructions and sinful ways become hindrances to God's healing and footholds for sickness and disease in our lives.

I have already given you specific scriptures which identify Jesus as our Healer (see page 90). Other Scriptures in the Bible describe the source of disease. You see, some people have the mistaken notion that God puts disease on us to teach us, to train us or to mature us. God doesn't do that. God does chastise and discipline His people. But He doesn't use disease to discipline us anymore than we teach our kids how to avoid fire by sticking their hands into a blazing furnace or hot oven.

The source of all illness is Satan. Jesus tells us very clearly that the devil has come to steal, kill and destroy (John 10:10). Jesus came to give us abundant life. God is the giver of good gifts — not evil gifts (James 1:12-17).

Our own destructions open the door to sickness and sin in our lives. Our own failures to take care of our bodies can lead to disease and illness. We need to ask God to use the Holy Spirit to reveal the destructions that we are bringing upon our own bodies. He will show us things that we are doing wrong. He will reveal any addictions or sin habits that open the door to Satan. When we understand that Jesus is the Healer, we will turn to His Word for revelation about all healing.

2. Inner peace is essential to healing.

The second principle that I share with my patients is the need to experience God's peace in preparation for our healing. Many people jump right in and start praying for their healing while their hearts are still full of fear, worry and anxiety. We must get rid of these things before we can experience God's peace in our lives.

> Be anxious for nothing, but in everything by prayer and supplication, with thanksgiving, let your requests be made known to God; and the peace of God, which surpasses all understanding, will guard your hearts and minds through Christ Jesus (Phil. 4:6-7).

This scripture tells us we can present our petitions to God. But before we pray we are to "be anxious for nothing"! We need to deal with the cares, worries and anxieties of our lives before we start praying. Often I tell my patients, "Don't start praying about this disease until you start dealing with your cares, worries and anxieties — then we'll pray!"

Some degree of anxiety and stress strikes all of us when our temples — our bodies — are threatened. God gave us the solution by saying, "Casting all your cares upon Him, for He cares for you" (1 Pet. 5:7).

You may wonder why you need to deal with the worry and anxiety. It is because anxiety will negate your faith. Fear, worry and anxiety counter your faith. We cannot walk in genuine faith and real peace as long as fear grips our lives.

We can deal with the fear, worry and anxiety by saying, "Lord, You told me to remember Your promises" (see Is. 43:26). You need to know and remember God's Word. Speak God's Word to your fear. Allow His perfect love to cast out all fear in your life. Peace will come with the remembrance of His Word.

3. Seek God's pathway of healing.

As you seek God concerning your pathway of healing, all you need is faith. Faith will bring healing.

Faith is not a tool of manipulation by which we force God to act as we desire. God sovereignly heals in His way, in His timing and with the pathway He chooses.

For example, heart disease strikes many people. God may heal one person through bypass surgery, another person through medication, others through balloon angioplasty, which opens up an artery in the heart with a balloon, and others through many other mechanisms. Still others may be healed supernaturally. It's time we began seeking God for His pathway of healing, rather than telling Him what we think He should do.

Seeking God's pathway rather than trying to manipulate Him to heal us according to our plan does not shut us off from the supernatural healing flow from God. Use the healing scriptures which you will find listed in Appendix A as you ask God, "What is my pathway to be healed? Which way am I to go? Is this the word of healing for me?" Then as God speaks to you, obey His leading.

The pathway of healing will always involve taking care of our bodies. For some, the pathway to healing will be through the use of medicine. At times the pathway will involve removing things that hinder our healing. Sometimes we may need to bind generational curses (see Deut. 5:9) so that genetic tendencies toward certain diseases will not be passed down in our families. Many times the pathway comes by taking antioxidants, vitamins and eating certain foods. I will talk more about this in the next section of this book.

4. The power of healing is available through the Holy Spirit.

The Spirit's power to heal indwells believers. That power

of healing has to be applied as the Holy Spirit reveals the pathway of healing. We can then lock onto the methods we are to follow. Once the woman who had suffered pain in her shoulders (see pgs. 40-41) started working through these spiritual principles of healing, she was entirely different. As she asked God to reveal her pathway to relieve pain, the Holy Spirit showed her a series of steps to follow. Then He gave her the power to follow His leading in her pathway of healing.

The story of the centurion's servant in the eighth chapter of Matthew demonstrated the power of healing in Jesus. The centurion recognized Jesus' authority and asked Jesus to speak the word of healing. He did not wait for Jesus to come to him. He sought Jesus out and activated his faith that Jesus would heal his servant. We activate our faith by authoritatively speaking God's Word to our problem (Mark 11:23). Are you speaking God's Word to your problem or illness?

We can also receive the power of healing through the prayer of agreement. "Again I say to you that if two of you agree on earth concerning anything that they ask, it will be done for them by My Father in heaven" (Matt. 18:19).

5. Be persistent in seeking your healing.

Healing is a process which often spans a period of time rather than involving an instantaneous, supernatural act by God. Yes, your healing can be instantaneous and supernatural, but it can also be a process requiring persistent prayer and overcoming faith that exercises patience. If God's pathway of healing for you is slow rather than go, can you wait on Him? James 5:13-18 tells of how we are to be persistent in our praying for healing. James points out that Elijah persistently prayed for three and one-half years before rain came. Going along patiently with God in our pathway of healing may involve weeks, months or even years. So be persistent in your prayer and faith for your healing.

When used alone, none of these five spiritual principles can lead to your healing. All of them work together as a whole to bring you to the source of your healing — Jesus Christ. Remember, a personal relationship with Him inspires you to love Him totally, listen to Him intently, obey His leading faithfully and take up your cross, following Him wherever He leads. Your healing was sealed on the cross and ultimately will be completed in heaven. Jesus is your Healer!

As we move into the part of this book where I share how God uses natural substances to guide us through our pathway of healing, you will discover:

- God's anointing can rest on natural substances.

- Nutrition, diet and natural things like herbs, vitamins and minerals can be used of God to treat and prevent disease.

- We can face the number one killer — cardiovascular disease.

- We can work toward the prevention of cancer and face it with spiritual authority and power.

- We can face other deadly diseases.

- How to choose the right doctor.

I am praying for you to move into the fullness of God's healing for you. Exercise your faith and begin to speak God's Word about healing. Cast on Him your anxiety, worry, fears and cares. Seek God for your pathway of healing. Let the power of healing spring from your spirit man through the indwelling Holy Spirit. Be persistent in your faith waiting on God for your complete healing through the Healer — Jesus Christ.

Chapter 8

DOCTOR and the WORD

WHY A CHRISTIAN *SHOULD* SEE A DOCTOR

Dr. Cherry, I'm a faith preacher," confided the pastor with the heart problem as he sat in front of me. "To be honest with you, this is a little frustrating to me...frankly, it's a little difficult for me to explain my illness to my congregation."

Is it strange for a Christian who believes in God's healing power to go to a doctor? I told this story in the previous chapter about this preacher who came to me for tests and treatment for his heart condition. He felt uncomfortable and somewhat embarrassed to share with his congregation his medical problems that needed treatment by a physician.

He did not have to feel that way. As we have discovered, God's pathway to healing may include both natural and supernatural means. Before I share specific areas of preventive medicine, let's review the important spiritual principles that we have already learned about our healing.

- God has a specific pathway that will lead to your healing.

- You must pray and seek God for that pathway

- God uses both the natural and supernatural to heal.

- All the healings that Jesus performed under that old covenant were effected on the basis of what He was going to do on Calvary when He established a new covenant.

- After you do what you can do in the natural, God will act in the supernatural to provide for your healing

- God provided a detailed plan of nutrition for His people.

- As a Christian, you have power and authority over disease through the blood of Jesus Christ

- You can take authority over sickness and disease in your body by seeing, reading, speaking and hearing God's Word.

Know the Natural Truth About God's Temple

There are some natural things you can do to be obedient to whatever God directs you to do in the natural for your healing. We are responsible for knowing the natural truth about the temple of the Holy Spirit — our bodies. A Christian physician can assist you in discovering what the Bible states about the care of your body.

The Bible clearly states that our bodies are the temple of the Holy Spirit, who indwells born-again believers

Do you not know that you are the temple of God and that the Spirit of God dwells in you? If anyone defiles the temple of God, God will destroy him. For the temple of God is holy, which temple you are (1 Cor. 3:16-17).

We are to be good stewards of all that God has given us, particularly of our bodies. Through us God acts and manifests Himself in the world. We are to be fit and healthy vessels for Him to use for His glory and purposes. Whatever destructive, sinful habits we have that harm our bodies need to be eliminated. Certain foods that we eat can do terrible damage to the temple of God. We cannot be a good witness for the God of the healing covenant, *Jehovah-Rapha,* when our bodies are being destroyed by our own destructive habits in the natural.

Learn all you can about your temple of the Holy Spirit, your body. Learn from a Christian doctor who knows about the body in the natural and who listens to the voice of God as he or she treats patients.

One of my responsibilities as a medical doctor is to share with you the best understanding that I have in the natural about your body. God gave us sound minds and keen intellects so that we can uncover the natural things which affect our bodies either positively or negatively. You need this understanding about God's design of your body, if for no other reason than to know how to pray.

Remember, no curse is causeless (Prov. 26:2). Sickness and disease are a curse. There are causes to the curse of disease in the natural realm as well as the spiritual attacks that the enemy uses to afflict us.

We should not be ignorant of the supernatural wiles or tactics of the devil (Eph. 6:11), nor should we be ignorant of the natural causes of disease. In His love and mercy, God has provided supernatural protection for us from the attacks of the enemy through His armor (Eph. 6). He has also provided a natural prevention for us to utilize so that we may head off and prevent many diseases. The following part of the book will highlight some of the provisions God has made for us to use in stemming the tide of heart disease, cancer and other diseases like diabetes.

We are "fearfully and wonderfully made" (Ps. 113:14). As believers, we need to learn how God created our bodies to operate. I have been amazed at the number of Christian patients I have met that were very ignorant of the most basic of their bodily functions. They lacked both an understanding of how they were created to function by God and of the things in the natural that affected their bodies adversely.

> I will praise You, for I am fearfully and wonderfully made; marvelous are Your works, and that my soul knows very well (Ps. 139:14).

Did you notice the truth revealed at the end of that? "And that my soul knows very well." Our souls are the residences for our minds, thoughts, knowledge and intellect. We can know much about our bodies that God knit together in our mothers' wombs (Ps. 139:13).

One source of knowledge about our bodies comes from reading books and periodicals about recent medical research. Another source available is a Christian physician who practices medicine with excellence and with a perspective shaped by God's Word and the Holy Spirit.

I do not have an answer for every medical illness. Nor do I know every solution for any one disease. For some conditions there is no known answer. No one source of natural information about your body is complete. Receive input from a number of truthful sources. Pray for the leading of the Holy Spirit. Seek God for a Christian physician to consult with you. Understand the spiritual principles for healing, both natural and supernatural.

Take all the information and advice you receive to the Lord. Make certain before you take any action that you have done the following: Line up your action with God's Word; repent of any destructive habits in your life; pray for the clear leading of the Holy Spirit; receive the best medical information available to you; and consult with a Christian doctor who listens to God's voice. Let God's peace be your guide to the pathway of healing you follow.

Don't stop or start any medication or medical treatment based on a quick decision made from reading this book or hearing from any other single source. Be persistent and patient to seek out God's clear and full revelation to you before entering your pathway of healing. I am praying for your complete healing through the stripes and shed blood of Jesus Christ so that you may live life in health and prosperity, becoming all that you can be for His glory.

Chapter 9

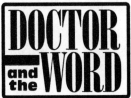

IS THERE A STONE
I MUST ROLL AWAY?

In an earlier chapter I discussed the story of Lazarus's healing (John 11). Jesus allowed Lazarus's mourners to do what they could do in the natural before He healed Lazarus supernaturally. Doing what we can do in the natural is "rolling away the stone."

Years ago my pastor, John Osteen, shared the following principle with me: There may be a stone you need to roll away before God moves, a natural action you can take to stop hindering God's healing power from working in your life. Rolling away the stone may require that you take a certain medication; go through a specific medical treatment such as surgery; undergo some form of medical therapy; or change your diet to help your body prevent disease.

Can I Follow Medical Treatment Plans and Still Stand in Faith for My Healing?

Taking medicine may be part of God's pathway of healing for you. Faith is not conditioned upon the use or nonuse of medication. Faith is trusting God for your healing — whether that means proper nutrition, exercise, taking medication or other natural steps. Let me illustrate this for you.

You may have been to doctor after doctor to try to find an answer to your suffering. You may know the Word of God. You may be standing in faith for your healing. You may have a clear understanding of what Jesus did on the cross to heal your body and your infirmities. Yet you may still be suffering.

I want you to ask this question, "Is there a stone that I need to roll away?" Specifically, I want you to ask yourself, "Am I following God's health and nutrition laws?" Now that may not be the entire answer, but it is often a starting point.

> Worship the Lord your God, and his blessing will be on your food and water. I [God] will take away sickness from among you, and none will miscarry or be barren in your land. I will give you a full life span (Ex. 23:25-26).

God Started With Good Nutrition

In Exodus 15:26, God introduced Himself as *Jehovah-Rapha,* the Lord God that heals thee. Then He began to introduce the subject of healing in the sixteenth chapter, beginning with nutrition. He discussed the methods for gathering and preparing food. As you discover God's plan for good nutrition, it will bring new life from His Word to you.

As you learn that God expects us to live a certain way according to his health and nutrition laws, you may recognize the destructive results in your body of not following these laws before now. You may have heart disease, hardening of the arteries or high blood pressure. Let's assume that the damage is already there. God has already made a way for you to get healed. God has created and anointed natural substances which have been uncovered in medical research.

Research has discovered that it is possible to reverse hardening of the arteries. How? We must first get blood fat levels as low as possible. This means that the total cholesterol level needs to drop below 170. As 170 and above levels are reached, fat that lines the arteries accumulates and begins to be reabsorbed into your system.

One of the first things a doctor should do is put you on a nutrition plan — one that lines up with God's Word in Genesis 1:29 where God talked about eating fruit and the fruits that bear seeds. Scientists today have discovered that certain seeds — namely oats, beans, dried beans and pintos — can lower your blood fat levels.

The world has gone full circle to the very beginning where God started this whole thing. Today, doctors are prescribing diets based on truths that God revealed in His Word.

For some, the blood fats may not come down as they should even on a strict diet. Is it hopeless? Has God suddenly run out of ways to heal you?

Let me tell you about another recent discovery. We have made an unusual discovery in medicine based on something that God created. Scientists have been researching a particular plant from which they have been able to isolate a chemical (compactin) which has been found to be the most potent chemical known to lower blood cholesterol levels. It could decrease cholesterol levels by more than half. This chemical is currently available by prescription (known as statin drugs) and is very safe. It has been shown to reverse hardening of the arteries and cut the incidence of heart attacks nearly in half. Would you take such a medicine if this were the stone you were to roll away?

In His Word, God said that He would satisfy us with long life and show us His salvation (Ps. 91:16). What a promise to His children! He has, in spite of our ignorance, misunderstandings or lack of knowledge of His health laws, made a way for His people to reverse the problem of hardening of the arteries. The answer is revealed through one of His created plants.

That is why you must be led by the Spirit of God to a doctor who will take the time to pray with you and seek an answer from God about the treatment for your particular situation.

God has given us a vast array of substances that He created and can use for our healing. He has also given us dietary laws. For example, God has now shown us another thing that has been hidden in nature for centuries. The Bible says God will give man "knowledge of witty inventions" (Prov. 8:12, KJV). I love that Scripture because it shows that great medical discoveries are inspired by an inquisitive mind that came from God.

You may say, "Well, I don't believe in medicine." Well, I don't either. I believe in the source of all healing — Jesus Christ. I don't like to use medicine. Yet, if it comes down to the choice of dying an early death or taking a pill that has a chemical that God created, what are you going to do? We can make a choice to live. If God directs us to use a medicine as part of the pathway of healing for a patient, we will use it. Many times God has led us to use medicine for healing. And we believe a patient will be ready to get off all medicine as healing becomes manifest.

Many times patients say, "I don't want to be on a pill."

"We don't want to have to put you on a pill," I respond. "But we are at the point where it is going to become dangerous if we don't do something now."

At times heredity is a factor. A patient may be exercising and following their dietary restrictions as closely as possible. But if they cannot get their cholesterol under control, fatty plaque is likely to build up in the arteries and cause blockage. Then they face surgery. Even if it's just a balloon angioplasty, no one wants to go through surgery. So it takes some understanding and assurance to get some patients to understand how God can use anointed natural substances for their healing.

Does Medicine Help God?

Jokingly, we sometimes ask, "Is taking medicine helping God?" God gave us the medicine, so God is actually helping us.

Other times people will ask me, "Dr. Cherry, if I use medicine, doesn't it mean I don't have faith."

"Do you brush your teeth?" I respond.

"Well, of course," they reply. "I brush my teeth. Everyone brushes their teeth."

"Well," I continue, "do you have faith to believe that God can take care of your teeth?"

"Why sure I do."

"Then, why do you brush them?" I ask.

They are contradicting themselves. Certainly God can care for our teeth supernaturally, but He has made us stewards over our bodies, the temple of the Holy Spirit. If God can use dentists, toothpaste and mouth rinse to care for our teeth through our actions, can't we use other substances such as medicines to help our bodies fight against and overcome disease if God so directs?

The point is this: We help God when we do what He gives us the ability to do in the natural. Was Moses helping

God when he picked up the staff and parted the waters? God told him to do that. But God did not act supernaturally until Moses did what he could do in the natural. God was the source of the power Moses used to part the waters and lead the people across. God was saying to Moses, "It's time to quit crying out to Me with your prayers. It's time to act!" (see Ex. 14:15).

That's exactly the attitude you need to have today. If you are suffering in your body, there is a time to pray and a time to take action. Find the stone you need to roll away.

You do what you can do.
God will do what you can't do.

On many occasions, God has directed me to use a medicine to treat a patient. I try to eliminate the medicine as soon as possible. But there are times when patients need a medication for longer periods of time because their medical problem is so advanced and serious due, perhaps, to ignorance of God's health laws. They may have eaten fatty foods for years, not walking according to God's design for their bodies. As patients understand how God designed us to work, they will often begin preventive measures to protect their bodies which will allow them to eliminate their medications.

As a Believer, Should I Go to a Doctor?

Many Christian friends and patients complain that their doctors pull out a prescription pad immediately after an exam and prescribe three or four medications. We are all irritated by that kind of approach. But there are times when we do have to use medication.

Some would say, "That's not walking in faith, Dr.

Cherry." Yet the Bible says that faith without corresponding action is dead or worthless (James 2:17).

Remaining ignorant is not faith. Faith acts upon the truths of God, trusting Him to provide a pathway of healing. Faith trusts God to reveal both the natural and supernatural ways He desires to heal.

How One Woman Rolled Away a Stone

A precious, Spirit-filled woman came to me who had been experiencing severe depression for more than ten years. She cried at the least provocation. She had been hurt by the remarks of people in the ministry, and she could not love or forgive. She couldn't deal with the bitterness in her heart.

She sat at my desk and told me her story of ten years filled with anger, bitterness, depression and tears. Before the depression started she had been a strong Christian woman. She knew the Word of God and prayed with authority and power. She knew the truth. Still, she was suffering terribly.

I prayed, "God, what in the world do we do now? She knows the Word of God."

God spoke to me about this case, saying, "The reason she can't get out of this depression is because she has clung too long to her anger, hate and bitterness. There is a chemical imbalance in her brain. She cannot even pray and receive My Word anymore."

I prayed, "Dear God, how in the world do I help a Christian who has gone beyond the ability to pray or receive the Word of God?"

Then God said, "She needs to get the chemical imbalance straight, and then I will heal her."

I explained the situation to her with compassion and love. I recommended that she see a specialist who could put her on medication, assuring her, "After eight weeks or so on this medication you will be normal. You will be able to work through the depression and your frustrations. You will be able to forgive because you will be functioning normally."

Using medication for just a short period of time could bring about her healing from ten years of pain and hurt. But if she didn't get help, it would be next to impossible to work through these things.

The woman listened to God's pathway of healing for her. The stone that needed to be moved away first was her need to undergo treatment and take medication for her chemical imbalance. The stone that she had clung to so long was her belief that God could only heal her supernaturally. Now He had revealed some natural things she could do for her healing. Once her stone was rolled away, she proceeded down her pathway of healing with the Lord.

You may ask, "Why did God do it that way? Why can't she just be prayed for and get deliverance?" Well God could have healed her that way, but He chose another pathway for her to follow. I did not choose the pathway of her healing — God did.

You don't need to worry about how God will heal you. If you're suffering and hurting from depression, heart disease or whatever illness, don't be concerned about how or when God heals you. Simply believe His Word that He will heal you.

Don't Be Concerned With God's Method

God may use the natural, the supernatural or a combination of both to lead to your healing. Don't seek His method; just seek the Healer, Jesus Christ.

God told me that if, after two months of medication, this depressed lady's chemical levels were normal, she could go off the medicine. She would be able to pray, apply the Word and be set free of this destruction of depression. God had outlined a simple pathway to her healing.

Don't Miss God's Pathway for Your Healing

If we aren't careful, we can miss God's pathway of healing for us. Find the stones that need to be rolled away and ask God to show you the natural ways to healing. Trust Him for His supernatural healing. Seek the Lord, praying, "What do I need to do, Jesus, to get healed? What is there in the natural that I need to do to get my healing?"

Don't try to manipulate God and misappropriate your faith. You cannot control how God will heal you. His sovereign will declares that you will be healed in His time, in His way and for His glory. Are you willing to pray, "Lord show me the pathway of healing that You have for me"?

If you'll start praying that way, God will speak to you in a way you may have never imagined. He may show you some things that astound you. But I have yet to see a patient who could not get healed if they were willing to listen to God and follow the path that He outlined for them.

Unbelievers miss God's healing pathway. Unsaved people think the solution rests with getting to a doctor. They have no other hope. They don't have the Word of God. They don't understand God's healing covenant with man. They don't understand the prayer of faith for healing. All they have are doctors. I would be seriously concerned if I had no one but a doctor to depend on. I can say that because I am a doctor, and I know how inadequate I am without the leading of the Holy Spirit. I am simply an instrument to be used by God for healing in the lives of His people.

The world takes natural healing to an extreme by rushing to the doctor, checking into the best hospital, finding the best specialists, taking all the medications or using surgical procedures that the world deems necessary for healing. By focusing solely on the natural without seeking God's pathway of healing, the world misses God.

Some Christians go to opposite extremes by believing that all healing must be supernatural. They say, "Well, bless God. I'm going to stand upon the Word, and I'm just going to wait in faith. If it's God's will, He's going to heal me." You have seen that kind of approach. It tries to manipulate God by trying to control the way and the time that He heals. God is sovereign. He will not be forced to heal us by contrived formulas or religious rituals.

I want you to see the balance. As you ask God to reveal the stone you need to roll away in preparation for His healing, He will reveal the path you are to take. It may be natural. It may be supernatural. It may be a change of attitude.

If you don't know how to pray for healing, God will help you. If you need to take proper steps for eating the right kinds of food and getting adequate exercise, He will reveal His plan. We will explore the topic of diet and proper nutrition in the next chapter.

Yes, you can use medicine wisely and consult a doctor. God can and does use the natural as well as the supernatural to heal. Take a moment now to ask the Holy Spirit to reveal God's pathway to you, identifying any stones that you need to roll away in preparation to follow His plan.

Chapter 10

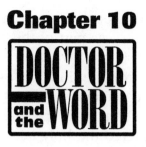

PREVENTING DISEASE WITH DIET AND EXERCISE

Believe it or not, what you eat affects your immune system as well as your entire body. You can help your body fight disease, or you can bring destruction to your body through what enters your mouth. The exercise you get, or fail to get, also affects your body — the temple of the Holy Spirit.

What Can I Do if I Dislike Exercise?

People protest all the time, "But, Dr. Cherry, it doesn't say in the Bible to exercise." Jesus did not tell people to exercise because people in His day already had an abundance of exercise. They walked every place they went, often twenty or thirty miles at a time. Jesus and His disciples walked from Galilee to Jerusalem and around Judea and Samaria. Exercise was part of the daily routine of life. Today some people simply have a hard time working exercise into their daily routine. But it is essential to maintain your body in good condition.

Exercise was abundant as the people of Israel walked in the desert or conquered the holy land with Joshua. Hard, physical work permeated everything done in ancient days. Think about wandering for forty years in the wilderness. Now that's getting aerobic exercise!

My wife, Linda, herself a nurse, is my partner in seeking just the right nutrition for both of us. But she doesn't enjoy exercise to the same degree I do. Still, both of us are exercisers — we just go about it differently. I usually run four to five miles several days a week.

Linda hates to perspire, but she has adjusted to it in order to exercise properly. We invested in a cross-country simulator that gives a good indoor workout for the arms, upper body and legs as well as the heart and lungs.

Running is difficult for many of our patients, so we put them on a walking regime, walking up to three miles in forty to forty-five minutes, five days a week.

Remember that observant Jews whom Jesus healed were functioning under old covenant health laws. They ate nutritiously and walked regularly — they had no other choice. It's very different now because we live in an industrialized country that has become very sedentary. We need to plan for exercise in our daily routines in order to keep our bodies fit vessels for the Lord to use.

A Good Reason to Exercise

I want to give you at least one reason why we put our patients on regular exercise. God created us in such a way that when we exercise regularly our level of HDL (high-density lipoprotein), a cholesterol-poor, protein-rich blood plasma, increases in our bodies. This is truly fascinating. God has built within men and women a way to reverse naturally the process of hardening of the arteries. A molecule of HDL is released when we exercise. This particle goes into our arteries, removing fat from the arteries and taking it to the liver where fat is excreted from the body.

People have a certain amount of HDL in their bodies. But due to our sedentary lifestyles, our HDL levels decrease significantly unless we exercise. As we exercise, HDL increases in our bloodstream and fat is carried away from our arteries and out of the body. For every one point that your HDL cholesterol increases, your risk of heart disease drops five percentage points. That's very significant.

Be careful to begin your exercise slowly, and increase the levels as you work out. Sudden exercise, or trying to do too much when you start exercising, can hurt your body. A treadmill stress test should be done before beginning an exercise program.

Can I Avoid Checkups if I Exercise?

Exercise does not guarantee health. We still must listen to God for our pathway of healing. What do I mean? Let me share with you this story.

As Linda and I sat in church one Sunday, God spoke to me. "I want you to get up in the middle of the service, go over to the gentleman halfway across the room and ask him about his health."

I said, "Dear God, how in the world can I get up in the middle of a service and do that?"

I told Linda. My wife, my wonderful encourager, asked, "Are you sure this is God?"

"Linda, this is God," I replied. "I must get up and go talk to that man."

Just as I stood up, the pastor said, "I feel a Spirit of praise. Let's stand and begin praising God."

Immediately God spoke again, "Go over there right now. I just made a way."

So I walked up to the man and asked, "How have you been feeling, Brother?"

"I've been feeling great," he responded.

"Have you had a physical recently?" I asked.

"Haven't had a checkup in years. I poured concrete yesterday. I do physical work all the time. I feel great," he assured me.

"I'll tell you what," I continued. "I think God wants you to pray about having a checkup. Go home and talk with your wife. Pray about it. If it's God, we'll both know it," I said.

In a few days, the man called the office and said he felt that God wanted him to have the checkup. He said the thought just wouldn't leave his mind. When he came to the clinic we ran extensive tests on him, but everything appeared to be normal. I thought, *God, what is going on here?* We checked his blood and his resting electrocardiogram. I listened to his heart and his lungs. Everything was checking out normally. The last test that we did that morning was a stress test to evaluate the arteries. We put him on the treadmill.

In the middle of the test, Linda called me and said, "You'd better get in here."

I rushed in and looked at his tracings. I could hardly believe my eyes. Every lead going to his heart was giving an abnormal reading. I said, "Brother, are you OK? How do you feel?"

"I feel great," he responded. "I could walk up here all day." He didn't have any pain! There was not a hint that anything was wrong. He kept walking until I finally took him off the treadmill. His test was very abnormal.

I told him, "We are seeing abnormalities, and we need to pray." God led us to get an angiogram. We took pictures of his coronary arteries and discovered that every major artery in that man's heart was totally blocked.

I asked him, "You poured concrete last Saturday and didn't feel any pain?"

He replied, "Never have felt any pain."

I couldn't believe that he had done such strenuous exercise and felt no symptoms. God had protected him.

So I prayed, "God, what are we to do now?"

God said, "His problem is extremely acute. I have protected him until now, but action has got to be taken right now." God directed us strongly to do bypass surgery.

A few days later he had the surgery. He recovered marvelously and was back pouring concrete in a few weeks. He had been sitting on a keg of dynamite waiting for a heart attack to occur even though he had plenty of exercise and appeared to be completely healthy.

That illustration shows us the way God worked on his behalf. God worked supernaturally, pointing out the problem in the middle of a church service; then God worked through another natural mechanism, bypass surgery, to open his arteries. He's healthier today than he has ever been. But he didn't sit around arguing with God about what to do. He heard from God, and I heard from God.

Even as he prepared for the surgery, he had the peace of God. What gives us peace is not exercise or staying physically fit. Going to the doctor regularly and having checkups will not give us true peace. Exercise and checkups are important. I believe God wants us to take care of our bodies for His glory. But our peace comes from hearing from God and doing what He asks us to do in the natural.

Are you listening to God for your pathway of healing? Are you exercising and keeping fit as He directs you? Are you caring for your body, His temple, the way He directs? As you listen to and obey the Lord, you will have great joy and peace as well as excellent health.

What About Dieting to Stay Healthy?

There is a trend these days toward dieting and exercising for health. We seem to be bombarded with advertisements and infomercials for various diet programs and exercise routines and equipment. God's perfect health plan as revealed in the Bible will guide us in the kind of diet we need. His health plan is not just a weight-loss plan. Rather, when we eat foods that God has provided for the prevention of disease and for the protection of our bodies, excess weight will not be a problem for us.

Remember the story of Naaman (2 Kin. 5)? Through His prophet, Elisha, God told this Syrian general to do something simple to be healed and returned to good health. He had to dip himself seven times in the Jordan River. At first Naaman was angry and unwilling to obey God. Yet that simple act of obedience brought healing and health to Naaman. He didn't like it. He thought it was stupid. Yet when He followed the leading of God, he was healed.

God has provided some simple ways to eat and take care of our bodies in the natural, but so many people seem to resist them. Yet these simple things can bring healing, health and protection to our bodies. I am going to share with you some very simple things about your diet and nutrition that will bring a multitude of health benefits to your life. Listen carefully to God's leading as you read through these simple things to do. Remember that we are to do what we can do in the natural. God will do supernaturally what we can't do.

Simple Nutrition Actions

The following suggestions will help you to take some simple nutrition actions which will help you to maintain good health.

1. Don't eat fat.

There are many things that can hinder your healing. We talked about some of these earlier in the book such as not walking in love and forgiveness. The way you think can hinder your healing. If your thoughts are not the thoughts of God, you hinder His Spirit from working in you. Inability to pray hinders your healing also.

Let's talk about some natural things that may be blocking your healing in the area of God's physical health laws.

The illustration we just used of the man with blockage of his arteries showed him to be a candidate for stroke, heart attack and serious health problems in his future. Approximately 53 percent of Americans die of blood vessel disease, heart attacks and strokes.

God knew we would face this situation thirty-five centuries ago when He outlined health laws to the Israelites. He talked specifically about fat in their diet. God forbade the eating of certain fats in His healing covenant.

> This shall be a perpetual statute throughout your generations in all your dwellings: you shall eat neither fat, nor blood (Lev. 3:17).

> Speak to the children of Israel, saying, 'You shall not eat any fat' (Lev. 7:23).

Nutrition plays a much more important role than we ever thought before in our healing. So many foods, especially the fatty foods, not only can clog up your arteries but they cause cancer. People come into our office all the time saying, "I have a great cholesterol — my cholesterol is 140. There's no heart disease in my family. I can get away with eating fat."

Fats not only clog up arteries but fatty foods are a major contributor to cancer. They weaken the immune system.

As we see a change in the dietary habits of Americans, Europeans and other industrialized countries toward eating more fat, the incidence of cancer goes up. Look at the major cancers that affect people in industrialized countries and notice the cause that scientists have determined.

While statistics constantly change, it's been reported that one American in fifteen now gets colon cancer. As I think back to the people I have treated with colon cancer, most were ignorant of God's nutritional laws. Perhaps they understood the Bible, having a good understanding of healing, faith and spiritual authority over disease. But they were ignorant of God's health laws. High fat and cholesterol intake puts us at high risk of prostate cancer (the number one cancer found in non-smoking males), endometrial cancer (cancer in the lining of the uterus or the womb) and breast cancer.

Eating fat puts people into a high-risk category for both cancer and heart disease. For the protection of our bodies, God plainly tells us: Don't eat fat. Violating God's basic health laws contributes to disease and hinders God's healing power in our lives.

2. Take vitamins and minerals to help your immune system.

Medical researchers have discovered that if a cancer patient has a viral or bacterial infection in his body that many times the cancer tumors disappear. Apparently the immune system is stimulated and stirred up by the virus or infection.

The number one stimulant to the immune system for believers is prayer. As you exercise your faith, God can bring substance to your healing (see Heb. 11). As you pray, your faith can give you substance (reality) to what you hoped for. But you don't have to get sick with a virus or bacterial infection to stimulate your immune system

When a person reaches his or her late twenties, the immune system begins to lose some of its effectiveness. It starts slowly going downhill unless we take corrective measures. Eating fat reduces the effectiveness of the immune system. But we can begin to stem the tide of a weakening immune system in one simple action.

Research has demonstrated that the immune system can be strengthened by taking multivitamins. The University of Medicine and Dentistry of New Jersey did studies on healthy men and women between the ages of 59 and 85. The researchers put patients on a simple multivitamin. They found that after one year of taking a multivitamin, their immune system responses soared approximately 64 percent. The T lymphocyte cells and antibodies sprang into action. Their potency increased with just a multivitamin. Even older people who were on good diets eating relatively low-fat foods had their immune systems stimulated when they took a multivitamin.

In the spiritual sense, the Bible speaks frequently of God placing a "hedge of protection" around His people (Job 1:10). In the natural, God has also created a "natural" hedge of protection inside the human body to protect us from a vast onslaught of disease and illness. This natural hedge is the immune system.

This incredible system protects us from anything — from the sniffles or a cold to the destruction of cancer. An overreactive immune system, on the other hand, can attack our own body cells, resulting in diseases such as lupus, rheumatoid arthritis and allergies (autoimmune diseases). A failure of the immune system can result in cancer. A weakened immune system accelerates the aging process.

Medical research has begun to discover a fascinating array of substances that actually strengthen the immune system. It turns out that God has already provided substances in the plant kingdom to enhance our immune function. We are now able to concentrate these substances and use them to build up our hedge of protection to fight off many diseases and illnesses.

The following is an overview to show how some of these vitamins and minerals can stimulate the immune system and help us fight disease naturally. You see, God has given us some simple things to do in the natural to protect and strengthen our bodies for His glory.

Vitamin E. Vitamin E is an enhancer of the immune system. Some studies call it a rejuvenator of the immune system function because it decreases any inherent weakness in the immune system. It can increase certain hormones that fight cancer cells and bacteria. We recommend 800 I.U. (international units) per day (capsule form) of natural, not synthetic, vitamin E. (The synthetic form is different chemically.)

Vitamin B. Vitamin B_6 can actually stimulate the lymphocytes that fight off infection and cancer. Some studies have suggested its use in the treatment of arthritis because it enhances immune system function. B_{100} complex contains all the various B vitamins.

Vitamin C. This vitamin is important to increase the number of white blood cells that form the backbone of our immune response. Take 1,000 mg of vitamin C twice daily.

Zinc. Zinc has long been known as an important substance in protecting the immune system. Too much, however, can cause harmful effects — 15 to 30 mg daily is sufficient.

Chromium. Chromium has an indirect effect on the immune system by stimulating T lymphocytes and interferon. Take 200 mcg daily.

Yogurt. The live cultures in yogurt stimulate the immune system by causing the body to increase production of gamma interferon which fights off infection. One to two cups daily (live culture) are recommended. Remember that frozen yogurt does not have live cultures.

Coenzyme Q-10. Studies show that this enzyme can increase an important component of the immune system (gamma globulin). 30 mg daily is recommended as maintenance therapy and 90 mg is recommended if disease is present.

Garlic. Garlic can stimulate and enhance the response of the immune system. Take the capsule form which is equivalent to one clove of fresh garlic daily.

Selenium. Selenium can enhance immune system function especially in fighting cancer. It can, however, be toxic in high dosages. Limit your intake to 100 mcg daily.

Echinacea. This plant substance can also stimulate immune system function. It should not be taken daily, as a tolerance can develop which could make it less effective. Take 2 to 3 teaspoons of tincture daily (or you can take the capsules) for four to eight weeks. Then stop taking it for two weeks.

Glutathione. Glutathione is a potent antioxidant and immune system stimulant. 100 mg daily is a standard dose.

3. Eat foods that fight disease.

There is so much more I could share with you about diet and nutrition. What I want to do in this book is to give you some simple ways to get started following God's health plan.

Eat foods that will help your body prevent and fight diseases. Some foods appear to be very effective at fighting diseases such as cancer and heart disease.

In Matthew 24, Jesus describes several events that will occur in the last days. In the seventh verse He specifically mentions *pestilences* (diseases). Many of the diseases we will see in the last days will attack our immune system. We must fortify and strengthen the immune system as much as possible.

Researchers have now identified many substances that strengthen the immune system and decrease the occurrence of many forms of cancer and heart disease. One such group is known as antioxidants. These include vitamin C, vitamin E, beta carotene and selenium. The following list shows foods that contain these important disease fighting substances:

1. Vitamin C: citrus fruits, strawberries, cantaloupe, broccoli, potatoes, tomatoes and other fruits

2. Vitamin E: vegetable oils, wheat germ, whole grain breads and pastas

3. Beta carotene: broccoli, cantaloupe, carrots, spinach, squash, pumpkin, sweet potatoes, apricots, other dark green, orange and yellow vegetables

4. Selenium: fish, lean red meat, breads and cereals

Another substance that seems to have a strong, protective effect on numerous body functions is the trace mineral chromium — found in brewer's yeast, whole wheat products, wheat bran, apple peel and other substances. Chromium plays a role in the prevention and treatment of diabetes, lowering cholesterol levels, fighting heart disease cataracts and may even help slow the aging process.

I urge you to eat right. Follow God's health plan for your body — the temple of the Holy Spirit. I would like to share some of the major diseases and health problems that we face in this country — heart disease, cancer and diabetes. God has given us some natural paths to follow that will help prevent and fight these terrible pestilences in our day. Continue reading for a more detailed examination of these diseases and discover ways that God has provided for their prevention and healing.

Chapter 11

DOCTOR and the WORD

FOODS THAT FIGHT DEPRESSION AND MEMORY LOSS

Our patients are constantly asking how they can improve or maintain their memories. Many patients seem to become forgetful as they get older or become more stressed or depressed in their lifestyles. Two things that affect our minds commonly are depression and memory loss. There are certain foods that you can eat which will help prevent memory loss and even enhance your present memory.

Overcoming Depression

The following foods contain God-created substances that seem to have a positive effect on depression.

1. Coffee

Coffee, which comes from a bean and contains caffeine, is the world's most widely used antidepressant. God has put it within man to seek out various things that can protect the mind and counter depression. Caffeine is a widely used mood elevator taken by millions of people. Studies show it can indeed function as a mild antidepressant through a complex effect on certain brain chemicals. Additional studies indicate caffeine can actually increase concentration, reaction times and thought processes. Don't exceed two cups of regular coffee daily. Certain people should avoid caffeine entirely (including those with irregular heartbeats or fibrocystic breast changes). Caffeine does not cause cancer or heart disease

2. Fish

For years we have called fish "brain food." Seafood is high in selenium, and studies have shown that people who do not get enough selenium in their bodies tend to suffer more depression, fatigue and anxiety. Selenium in fish also protects against cancer

3. Nuts

Certain nuts such as almonds and Brazil nuts are very important to a healthy diet. Brazil nuts, sunflower seeds and oat bran are all high in selenium

4. Garlic

Garlic literally kills cancer cells. It also has a mood-elevating property. Studies done in Germany have found that people suffering from depression were less fatigued, anxious and irritable after taking garlic preparations.

Garlic supplements are widely sold overseas and are more available in this country than they were a few years ago. One lady who is a patient of our clinic chops garlic and eats it raw. I asked her, "Don't your friends comment about your breath?"

"Oh yes," she replied. "They do. They say I stink all the time."

"So what do you tell them?" I asked.

She said, "I tell them it's healthy, and if you don't like me being healthy, you know, that's your problem. But I'm going to eat it."

Well, very kindly I shared with her a better way to get enough garlic by taking concentrated supplements which are readily available.

God, in His wisdom has blessed our food by choosing particular compounds for multiple protection. Many times the Bible talks about leeks and onions and garlic. The mention of garlic appears over and over again in God's Word. We are now recommending garlic supplements to the patients we are treating for heart disease, cancer, as well as to those who want to feel better emotionally.

Before you begin to take any substance, pray about it. God may restrict you from taking certain substances. Something in your body may not agree with garlic or another substance. Always be sensitive to the leading of the Spirit.

5. Peppers

Another food helpful in the treatment of depression is chili peppers. Chili peppers increase the level of endorphins in the brain. Endorphins elevate mood. Did you know that some people get hooked on chili peppers, eating stronger and stronger chili peppers because of this endorphin release? The peppers really make them feel better.

Enhancing Memory Function

There are also foods you can eat that enhance your

memory function. Memory is a major concern to many of our aging patients. It is not unusual for an older adult to forget names and small details. We need to identify natural ways that God gave us to keep our minds sharp. Let me share five substances with you that help your memory.

1. Zinc

Slight deficiencies of zinc in your body can lead to poor memory function and slower general mental activity. Regular intake of cereal, turkey and legumes (all high in zinc) can prevent zinc deficiencies. The amount of zinc in most multiple vitamins is sufficient to supply our needs.

2. Carotene

Adequate amounts of carotene are critical to insure proper thought processes. Good sources of carotene are dark green, leafy vegetables, carrots and sweet potatoes. One 15 mg capsule taken daily can supply more than enough carotene for your intake. Carotene also gives some cancer and heart protection as well.

3. Iron

Iron is essential for normal mental function. Iron can be found in green vegetables, lean red meats and in multiple vitamins. Remember, excessive amounts can be harmful.

4. Riboflavin

Riboflavin is found in almonds (ten a day), cereals and skim milk. This B-complex vitamin helps memory function.

5. Thiamin

Another essential substance for normal memory function, thiamin, is found in wheat bran cereal, nuts and wheat germ.

Avoiding animal fat is also essential in enhancing memory function. Fat can alter the function of chemical transmitters in the brain. That, in turn, causes memory changes and affects thought processes. Eat lean beef no more than once weekly. Remember that it is possible to lower fat consumption by substituting skim milk (or even 1 percent or 2 percent milk) for whole and using fat-free cheeses. Consume very few sweets (or none at all), very little butter or margarine, and remove the skin from poultry.

A pastor from a northern state who had suffered from depression for over twenty years called our clinic and told us he had never had a really joyous, happy time since the sixth grade. Because he lived so far away, I was reluctant for him to spend the time and money to come to the clinic when we had treated so few people with depression at that time.

However, he was very eager to come. I could hear the desperation in his voice as he said, "You are my last hope!"

When someone says that, I reach out to the Lord and say, "Lord, tell me what to say to this man. Tell me whether to encourage him to come or whether to discourage him. Should I tell him to get to a psychiatrist who could prescribe medication?" He had been reaching out for help for years, and he had spent much time praying for God to reveal His will about his depression.

He was willing to make the journey of faith to get the help he needed. When he arrived I checked him over to find out if there was a problem. God led us to the medication that he needed to take, which was a new class of medicines.

I didn't hear God clearly at first. I knew God was telling me to use the new medicine, but I could not recall the name of the medicine because it was so new. I suggested that he return home.

"No, Dr. Cherry," he insisted. "God is going to speak to you; don't give up on me."

I prayed again, "God, I know there's a drug to use. Please help me to recall its name."

God brought to mind the name of the right medicine, and we gave it to this pastor. After a short period of time he called me, "This is the first time I have laughed since the sixth grade," he exclaimed. "This is the first time I have whistled to myself since then. God has touched me and restored those chemical levels to normal." He went on to tell me that he used to whistle when he was a little boy when he was happy. It was a simple pleasure he had not been able to enjoy for years. Now he was whistling again.

Ask God to show you what will help you with your own depression or memory loss. Through natural substances, God has given us foods that will fight depression and memory loss. Take action now to include these foods in your diet in order to care for your body — the temple in which His Spirit dwells.

Chapter 12

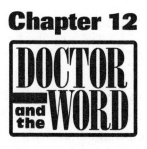

FOODS THAT FIGHT HEART DISEASE

Th
here are approximately sixty million cases of high blood
pressure (hypertension) that occur in this country annually.
High blood pressure contributes to heart disease and
strokes, as well as causing the blockage of blood vessels
(peripheral vascular disease) in the legs and extremities.
Hypertension can ultimately lead to renal disease or kidney
failure. But what I want to emphasize to you is God's provision. God has designed a human body to function
without the use of pills and medication in order to take
care of us and to protect us from high blood pressure. Let's
look at some of these ways.

High blood pressure is one of the main contributors to
heart disease. But God has provided some amazing natural

substances which can help reduce heart disease. God has given us certain things we can do in the natural for our protection and health

> I call heaven and earth to record this day against you, that I have set before you life and death, blessing and cursing: therefore choose life, that both thou and thy seed may live (Deut. 30:19, KJV).

One of the things that I see in this particular scripture is that when God lays life before us, He is also laying before us His health laws. God has indeed made a provision to take care of His people. This applies to all the areas of our lives including the major diseases that affect us in this day and age.

In this chapter we will primarily explore a particular aspect of heart disease which has become the silent killer — high blood pressure (hypertension). When I was in medical school the primary way we had to deal with blood pressure was through medication. In fact, for decades the major thrust of the way doctors have treated high blood pressure is to take a prescription pad and put people on pills. It's amazing to see all the articles in major medical journals that have appeared in recent years regarding hypertension and ways of treatment in the natural.

Yet God has given us some excellent natural ways to protect against and treat high blood pressure.

1. Weight reduction

Sometimes when I talk about weight reduction, some people throw their hands in the air. They feel as if they have to lose a lot of weight before they can experience any positive health effects — not true. Studies show that with as little weight loss as four to eight pounds, blood pressure can drop significantly, even as much as eight to ten points. That's such a simple but important thing to do in the natural

2. Calcium

Calcium can help to protect against colon cancer. Calcium also has a protective effect on us for heart disease. Studies have also shown that calcium often reduces high blood pressure when other elements do not.

When an intake of 450 to 600 milligrams of calcium a day was given to the individuals taking part in one study, only 9 to 12 percent of the group continued to show high blood pressure. When the calcium intake increased to 1,200 to 1,400 milligrams daily, only 3 to 6 percent of the group registered high blood pressure. God has given a provision or protective effect against hypertension with calcium.

Dairy products are one of the ways we suggest patients get their calcium requirements. For example, drink skim milk (or 1 percent or 2 percent), and include foods in your diet such as low-fat cottage cheese and low-fat yogurt, both of which are excellent sources for calcium.

Calcium supplements are also available and are especially useful when patients cannot tolerate dairy products in their diets. But if you are going to consume a calcium supplement, you need to do it on an empty stomach. Calcium is very poorly absorbed in situations where gastric acid is diluted. So we need to consume calcium early in the morning when it is absorbed easier. Up to 1,200 milligrams daily is generally recommended because of the effect it can have to lower blood pressure.

3. Potassium

Potassium has also been associated with a drop in blood pressure. This is another anointed substance in the natural that God has provided. Studies have shown that 40 percent of the daily potassium in the American diet comes from dairy products. Many fruits, such as bananas, have higher levels of potassium, as do many vegetables.

4. Avoid saturated fat

The countries in the world that lead the world in coronary and artery disease are high consumers of fatty foods, one of which is butter. Even margarine can cause problems. There is really no contest between butter and margarine. Butter contains 54 percent of saturated fat, whereas there is only 18 percent of saturated fat in margarine. So margarine is less harmful (olive oil would be better than either, however). Every major researcher in cancer as well as heart disease recommends monosaturated fats over saturated fat. The key is to look at total fat content. Fat calories should be no more than 20 percent of your total calories.

God's Natural Ways to Fight Heart Disease

The largest contribution you can make to reduce your risks of heart disease is to reduce fat intake. Statistics indicate that as many as 53 percent of Americans die from heart disease because of high blood pressure, stroke, heart attacks and congestive heart failure. The following steps can be taken to reverse heart disease if you have it or to prevent it if you are free from problems now. Thank God that He has given us some of these natural things we can do to fight this terrible curse.

1. Reducing fat intake

I know this may sound like a broken record, but it is so important. Here are some ways to reduce fat intake:

- Eat beef no more than once a week.

- Use olive oil and canola oil for cooking.

- Eat no meat at all three days a week, eating only fruits and vegetables (rice, beans, pasta, baked potato, squash, broccoli, and so forth) on those three days.

- Eat fish at least two to three times a week (preferably cold water fish such as salmon, cod and herring).

2. Getting regular exercise

Exercise three to six times a week for thirty to sixty minutes continually each time so that your heart rate stays elevated. Walking, running, cycling, using exercise machines and swimming are all effective aerobic exercise for your heart.

3. Taking vitamins

Use a multivitamin daily, including 800 I.U. of vitamin E, 1,000 mg of vitamin C twice daily, 30 mg of beta carotene and 30 mg of B_{100} complex daily.

4. Coenzyme Q-10

Take 30 mg daily of coenzyme Q-10 (more with certain heart problems like congestive heart failure). Consult with your doctor.

5. Alcohol and tobacco

Keep alcohol intake very low in your diet. High amounts increase blood pressure and risk of stroke. Many studies have linked smoking to increased risk for both heart disease and cancer. Stop smoking. For many patients, using a nicotine patch can be very helpful. Check with your doctor.

6. Bran and fiber

Increase your intake of bran and fiber, especially water-soluble bran such as oat or wheat, to one-half cup daily.

7. Salt

Limit salt in your diet. Salt causes your body to retain fluids and may increase your blood pressure. Use "lite salt" or a salt substitute.

8. Complex carbohydrates

Eat more complex carbohydrates such as those found in fruits, cereals and vegetables. Go back to chapter 5 on nutrition for a review

9. Cholesterol

Get your cholesterol down. If eating a healthy diet doesn't lower your cholesterol, check with your doctor. There are some new, once-a-day medicines derived from plants that can lower cholesterol and reverse hardening of the arteries. One or two teaspoons of psyllium daily is also useful for lowering high cholesterol

10. Baby aspirin

Take one baby aspirin daily after checking with your doctor. Some people cannot take aspirin.

11. Regular checkups and controlling blood pressure

Get regular checkups. Seeing your doctor for regular stress tests, blood work and a good, head-to-toe physical is important. It is imperative to check your blood pressure regularly and keep it under control

12. Controlling blood sugar

If blood sugar is high, there are simple ways to lower it. See our discussion of diabetes in chapter 9.

13. Treating your symptoms

If you have symptoms such as angina (chest pain, tightness, pressure) or other signs of a change in health, don't ignore them. Check with a physician. Don't assume that pain, for example, is only indigestion. Be aware of changes in your body.

14. Trying garlic

One or two concentrated capsules a day thins the blood and raises HDL, which is good for your arteries.

We saw a patient at our clinic whose blood pressure was averaging about 160 over 105. We put him on the treadmill and his blood pressure shot up to over 230. Linda called me into the room so we both could monitor him closely. We prayed about what to do with him, and God led us to prescribe an ACE inhibitor — one little pill a day. By the afternoon, his blood pressure was 120 over 70. The patient said, "Dr. Cherry, I have never felt better. I didn't remember what it was like to feel so good."

High blood pressure can really pull you down and make you feel fatigued and drowsy. I told this man, "The day is going to come — we'll believe and pray for this together — that you will be off this medicine. If you lose the weight we talked about, get exercise, change your diet and limit your salt, I think you will be able to go off the medicine."

It's interesting to note that when God talks about His provisions in the Bible, God states that He is leading His people to the Promised Land — "the land of milk and

honey." Both milk and honey are filled with health benefits, and the land itself was overflowing agriculturally with
the production of fruits and vegetables. God was giving
them a land that could produce the foods they needed to
eat in order to live according to His health laws. Abounding
in Palestine were substances that God was actually giving
to His people to protect them from cancer, high blood pressure and heart disease.

If you have been diagnosed with high blood pressure, I
encourage you that there are many doctors today who will
give their patients a trial of diet and exercise before auto-
matically putting them on a medicine. We've been very
successful with many patients following this approach. In
fact, many of them have been able to discontinue their
blood pressure medicine if they are able to follow these
provisions.

Remember, do not change anything you are presently
doing without consulting your doctor. But consider the
things I have mentioned. Pray about them and suggest
them to a Christian physician.

Remember God's challenge: "I have set before you life
and death, blessing and cursing: therefore choose life"
(Deut. 30:19, KJV). The choice often centers around
whether you choose life by following His health laws or
you go another route. Your choice can determine the incidence of health problems you experience.

Like the man with high blood pressure, many Christians
can take control over their flesh and reverse the effects of
high blood pressure if they will do what they can do in the
natural. I like to encourage our patients not to be locked
onto the idea of taking a medicine. I can recall many
patients who are totally off their medications because they
have worked with a doctor and lined up with the Word of
God.

He who does not use his endeavors to heal him-self is brother to him who commits suicide (Prov. 18:9, AMP).

Don't just sit back and take life and good health for granted. Health is something you can vigorously seek. We need to diligently seek the path to total healing in our lives.

Chapter 13

DOCTOR
and the WORD

FOODS THAT FIGHT CANCER

Have you ever heard of mung beans? I knew nothing about mung beans until our research into ways to prevent cancer uncovered a chemical contained in these beans called ginseng — one example of a natural substance that God has created for our health and the prevention of disease.

Fighting Cancer

You can eat certain foods that will strengthen your immune system, fight cancer and help prevent illness. Here is a simple overview of some of these foods.

1. Ginseng

Mung beans look like tiny peas. They contain a chemical called ginseng that limits the blood supply to cancer cells. Cancer is on the increase — particularly colon cancer and breast cancer. A cancer has to have a strong blood supply because it grows so rapidly. In these beans, as well as in soy products, God gave us certain chemicals that literally shut off the blood supply to the cancer. Isn't that incredible? Mung beans are very low in fat and high in fiber They are especially good when served with rice.

To prepare mung beans, wash them and cover them with water, soaking them overnight in the refrigerator, or soak them five to six hours at room temperature. Pour the beans into a saucepan, bring to a boil and simmer until tender. Drain the beans and cook them until done.

This bean is used extensively in Asian diets, which may be a significant factor in the low cancer rates found among the Asian population.

2. Tea

Teas, specifically green tea, are consistently associated with a cancer protective effect. There are many different kinds and varieties of tea. It is not the herbal teas that are being studied in the realm of cancer prevention but rather the nonfermented green teas now available at many grocery stores.

Green tea contains a chemical that prevents cancer cells in the body from dividing. That's one reason people in Asia who drink four to five glasses of green tea a day have much lower rates of cancer. Studies in Shanghai and other parts of China show that one group of tea drinkers cut their risk of esophageal cancer (a very deadly cancer) by one-half compared to a group who was not drinking green tea.

3. Tomatoes

There is a potent chemical in tomatoes called lycopene (which gives them their redness). This chemical tends to protect the DNA in cells. Studies conducted in Italy found that people who ate raw tomatoes seven times a week cut their risk of a variety of cancers in half. A 50 percent reduction! This red pigment (lycopene) is found in many different plants, including watermelon, red peppers, carrots and strawberries. Lycopene is potent against prostate cancer.

4. Licorice root

The chemical in licorice root that makes it sweet is very effective in the prevention of prostate cancer. How do you use it? It often comes in small sticks. Use licorice sticks in a cup of tea to sweeten it. Incidentally, another plant called saw palmetto contains a chemical that can help shrink the enlarged prostate — a very common problem in men.

5. Citrus fruits

Oranges have shown strong anti-cancer benefits. Some sixty cancer-fighting chemical agents are found in citrus products. Many studies have also been conducted on grapes to demonstrate their strong effect in combating cancer.

6. Garlic and onions

Garlic and onions are being studied extensively because they have a cancer-protective and cancer-fighting effect. Over thirty anti-cancer compounds are present in these vegetables. Consider taking a dried garlic extract capsule (the equivalent of one clove) per day. Eat onions frequently in your diet.

7. Greens

The darker the greens, the better. Some of the cancer fighting agents in greens are lutein, beta carotene and carotenoids. Good sources of these agents are found in spinach, lettuce and broccoli.

8. Soybeans

These contain strong anti-cancer compounds (protease inhibitors, saponins) that increase immune system function Tofu, soy milk and other soy products are excellent.

Dietary Suggestions to Fight Cancer

If you have cancer and are fighting the disease, consider the following food and nutrition guidelines:

- Decrease, if not eliminate, animal fats
- Avoid safflower, corn and peanut oil
- Use more monounsaturated fats (olive oil, canola oil)

Increase your intake of the following:

- Garlic
- Fish oil

  Omega-3 fatty acids in cold water fish (cod, mackerel, herring) may decrease the size of cancerous tumors. Fish oil capsules may also be taken.

- Beta carotene

  This agent both prevents and fights cancer. Eat orange and yellow vegetables (such as sweet potatoes and cantaloupe). Use 15 mg of beta carotene per day, taken with other vitamins

- Cabbage and broccoli

  These vegetables are potent cancer fighters (especially for breast cancer)

- Yogurt

  Nonfat yogurt can help the body increase the level of cancer-fighting chemicals (gamma interferon). Eat six to eight ounces daily.

- Licorice

  We mentioned this earlier as an effective cancer fighter.

Remember, God has given us a multitude of foods (Gen. 1:29) to fight and prevent cancer. Eat right to care for your temple of the Holy Spirit. Combine your nutritional changes with an authoritative prayer life. You can have victory over all disease!

Chapter 14

DOCTOR and the WORD

FOODS THAT FIGHT DIABETES

It's incredible that five hundred thousand people develop diabetes every year in this country. It's been estimated that up to fifteen million Americans have diabetes.

The first stage of diabetes is what we call "glucose intolerance." One of the tests that we do at the clinic (often omitted in medical checkups) is a two-hour glucose tolerance test in which the patient drinks a measured dose of glucose. This kind of test can show us if a patient has a future tendency to develop diabetes.

There are some new findings that have come out that indicate we may be able to reverse diabetes. As Christians, we need to be aware of this new research. Sugar diabetes affects the nerves in the extremities, the arteries that go to the heart and to the kidneys, and our eyes, at times causing blindness. It's one of the world's leading causes of blindness. When I was in medical school the traditional thinking was to lower high blood sugar by limiting the intake of carbohydrates. A low-carbohydrate, high-protein diet for diabetes was advocated.

Much of that thinking has changed. Research has recently indicated that the way to treat diabetes is with a high-carbohydrate and low-fat diet (see Gen. 1:29 and Lev. 3:17).

Let's take a look at the two types of diabetes. Type II, the more common type of diabetes, may or may not require insulin but develops later in life, particularly if you gain weight. By going on certain high-fiber supplements (psyllium, bran), many Type II diabetics are able to go completely off their medications. It often takes only twenty days to do so. Remember, consult with a knowledgeable, Christian physician and follow God's direction for making these changes in your diet or medication.

The tougher form of diabetes, Type I diabetes, includes patients who are insulin dependent. Using certain diets, they are frequently able to reduce their dosage of insulin by 30 to 40 percent. Sugar levels typically drop in patients with Type I diabetes from 161 to 135, which is normal. The cut-off for normal is a blood sugar level of 140. Anything above that is considered to be diabetes.

When going on the type of program that I outline, the cholesterol levels may drop 25 to 30 percent, which is phenomenal. While we are trying to lower blood sugar levels, we are often able to lower the blood fat levels as well.

The diet combination I recommend also often lowers blood pressure by 10 percent. Another benefit is weight loss. The higher fiber tends to cause an increased expansion of the stomach, and people eat less. It also triggers certain enzymes in the intestines which tell the brain that the stomach is full. Wouldn't it be wonderful if we just felt full most of the time and didn't get so hungry? That's really the battle we face when fighting the urge to eat. The type of diet that we are working on with diabetes tends to do that.

Keys to Lowering Diabetic Risks

There are four major ways to lower your risk of diabetes and possibly reverse it if you already have it.

1. Water soluble fiber

Eat oat bran, consuming about one-third cup daily. Also eat dried beans (kidney, pinto and great northern beans), one-half cup five times weekly. Take psyllium, one to three teaspoons daily.

2. Fish

In a study carried out over a period of four years, 45 percent of people who did not eat fish developed glucose intolerance versus only 25 percent of the fish eaters. Cod, salmon, herring and trout tended to show the best results. I recommend eating at least one ounce of fish four to five times weekly.

3. Exercise

Get at least thirty minutes of continuous exercise three to four times a week. In one study those who exercised five or more times weekly had only 42 percent of the diabetes of those who exercised less than once weekly. Those exercising two to four times weekly had 38 percent less incidence of diabetes compared to those who exercised less than once weekly. Even those only exercising once weekly had 23 percent less incidence of diabetes compared to those who exercised less than once weekly

4. Vitamins and minerals

I recommend the use of a good multivitamin and mineral daily. Certain vitamins such as the antioxidants (vitamin C, beta carotene and selenium) may offer protection to the arteries of those who have diabetes. Chromium, in doses as high as 600 to 800 mcg daily, dramatically lowered blood sugar levels.

In my family several relatives had diabetes. I thank God I have normal blood sugar levels, but Linda and I both include these four things in our diet to help prevent diabetes. We are doing what we can do.

Do what you can to protect yourself from these diseases. God outlined the health and nutritional laws for us in His healing covenant so that we could follow our pathway of healing. Do what you can do in the natural, and God will act in the supernatural for your healing.

One man practically forced his wife to come to our clinic because he was so concerned about her. This woman never went back to the doctor after first being diagnosed with diabetes and receiving initial treatment.

She had not seen a doctor for ten years but had initially been put on insulin for two years. In faith she took herself off insulin, and for eight years she avoided medical care. She had a history of elevated blood pressure but also took herself off blood pressure medication. She had lost sixty pounds and was feeling extremely weak. She had partial paralysis in her left leg. Still, she did not consult a physician. Then while she slept she started having severe pains in her legs. For several months before visiting our clinic, she experienced excessive fatigue and occasional numbness in her left arm and left leg as well as a marked increase in her thirst. Nevertheless, she did not want to go to the doctor. Finally her husband insisted on bringing her to the clinic.

We examined her thoroughly and found that she had

exceptionally high levels of fasting blood sugars. Her two-hour glucose tolerance blood test was critically high. She had to be put back on insulin. Her condition had resulted in severe damage to several blood vessels and to numerous organs in her body because of her high sugar count. The blood vessels in the back of one of her eyes were damaged. She had major circulation problems and muscle atrophy in her lower extremities due to the diabetes.

The lesson to learn from her experience is this: Don't be ignorant about your body and how it functions. If you believe that God wants you to follow a different pathway of healing than the one you are now on, pray, seek God's Word, and be under the careful supervision of your doctor to get information about your body.

Diabetes is a terrible disease that has to be monitored regularly with blood tests. If someone is on insulin, they need to have insulin checks quite regularly. There are two sides to this whole thing. Yes, some people are healed of diabetes supernaturally. I have seen this several times. They never have it again. There's no medical explanation for it — it's a sovereign act of God. For others though, their pathway of healing involves using natural means to walk in their healing. Again, God has designed a path for each individual to follow that leads to his healing.

Seek God's Pathway of Healing for You

Remember the steps to healing which the blind man in the ninth chapter of John had to take with Jesus' help? Although Jesus put clay mixed with saliva on the man's eyes, healing was not manifested when Jesus touched him — an important and often overlooked point. He was only healed when he did as Jesus commanded him to do in the natural and washed in the pool of Siloam.

This principle shows you a new direction to pray for your healing. Pray, "Father I come to you in faith in the name of Jesus. Reveal to me the pathway that leads to my healing. Show me the steps to follow."

Remember that in many cases God uses your endeavors combined with your faith in the supernatural power of God to bring healing. God's pathway may not be completely in the natural or in the supernatural for you. Rather it may be a combination of both.

Although at times a person may *feel* as though he or she has been healed during the emotion of a service, you don't get healed with your head or your feelings. You may *feel* good. You may be caught up in the emotions of the moment. But the healing has to come out of your spirit man where God's Spirit dwells. And once it does that, my friend, it's all done. You are healed.

Just because you confess or believe that you are healed doesn't mean that God has acted. Don't be tempted to do foolish things when you just feel healed. I've had many patients who thought they were healed do foolish things. Sometimes it takes near heroic means to bring them back from disaster. That's why I encourage and stand in agreement with everybody to find God's pathway.

Remember, when you've done all you know to do, stand firm (Eph. 6). Doing what you can do in the natural does not mean that you do not trust God. There is no stigma for a Christian who takes medication or has surgery. God may use these things until we get our body lined up with His Word. The key is to let God reveal His pathway of healing!

Read my epilogue to experience the revelation of how one of the greatest healing evangelists of our time discovered God's pathway of healing for him — including both prayer and natural means.

Epilogue

DOCTOR and the WORD

GOD'S PATHWAY TO HEALING FOR ONE EVANGELIST

Yes, even a healing evangelist sometimes has to seek a pathway of healing from God. In the mideighties, a dear friend in Christ, Brother R. W. Shambach, faced a critical problem with his heart. He became my patient, and we walked together through his incredible pathway of healing.

Throughout this book, we have discussed how God uses both the natural and the supernatural for healing. It can be particularly difficult for a pastor, preacher or evangelist who preaches the supernatural healing power of God to face illness in his own life. At times, God may even use an evangelist who suffers from physical illness in his own body as an instrument of supernatural healing in the life of another person. It is possible for a man of God to seek

God's pathway of healing and discover that God can use both the natural and the supernatural to prevent and heal disease.

The following dialogue with Brother Shambach took place on our television program, *The Doctor and the Word*. I want you to read the words of Brother Shambach because what he has done is unique. He combined his faith with the power of prayer. The Bible says, "The spirit of man will sustain him in sickness" (Prov. 18:14). Brother Shambach demonstrated the above verse along with another scripture in Proverbs 18: "He who does not use his endeavors to heal himself is brother to him who commits suicide" (v. 9, AMP).

This is the solution. We exist in a natural body; we are not angelic beings. We do not exist in supernatural form. The Bible says we are vessels of clay (2 Cor. 4:7). So we're subject to physical laws. The key is to combine what God would have us do in the natural with God's supernatural power at work through faith and prayer.

Dr. Cherry: When you were under God's anointing, you really felt no symptoms in your body, did you?

Bro. Shambach: It's almost like a false security. You don't live in that anointing all the time. The Bible says, "Many are the afflictions of the righteous: but the Lord delivers him out of them all" (Ps. 34:19). A lot of times the only way you know you are in the will of God is the adversity that you are facing. If you don't have adversity, then you had better check up to see whether you are in the will of God. And thank God for the trials that come, and thank God when they go.

Dr. Cherry: Thank God more when they go than when they come!

Bro. Shambach: Amen.

Dr. Cherry: *[To the audience]* Brother Shambach's story of the attack on his body goes back to the 1980s when we first discovered a blockage in the arteries that go into his heart. Linda and I stood with him and his wife, Winn, and we set ourselves to seek the will of God and to find the pathway to his healing. Well God gave us a clear directive to go in and get those arteries opened up. Surgery was directed by God, and afterwards Brother Shambach felt terrific. Of course, the great call on his life was to go out and preach to all the world, and he did that. After surgery, his heart was strong, and he felt good.

You launched right back like you did before, didn't you, Brother Shambach?

Bro. Shambach: Same hectic pace. However, you put me on a regimen of proper nutrition. That's the most difficult thing for a preacher. When you are feeling good you say, "Man, I can eat anything I want now." You see, when you are under the anointing, and it's a heavy anointing when you are ministering to people, you feel like you can do anything, and you disregard your physical body. I have laid hands on people who were healed of heart disease — so many, I mean thousands of them. And that's the trick of the devil — to get you into a situation like that when you feel so strong under the anointing that you are tempted to change your eating habits. When you are feeling good, then you go back to bad habits that hurt your body. But I lost close to forty pounds this time. And I tell you, thin looks good. And I'm going to stay there. Salt was a challenge for me, though.

Dr. Cherry: Salt is an enemy because of fluid retention. If your heart gets weak and has trouble pumping, the last thing in the world it needs is more fluid. Salt pulls fluid into your body. You know how you put salt on a wound and it hurts? It hurts because it's pulling the fluid out of that tissue.

[To the audience] Well Brother Shambach went back on the road following a heavy schedule. Like he says, as a

preacher the meetings are often at night, so eating late at night after a meeting is so tempting. We've talked about how hard that is on the body.

But slowly the disease — Satan's attack — came back. Brother Shambach called me and said, "I need to see you. I think I need to get something checked in my body." He came to the clinic, and we examined him. His heart muscle was not beating like it should. It was extremely weakened to the point that it was technically called heart failure. That doesn't mean you are dying. It just means the pump is not working like it should.

I looked at that situation and said, "Brother Shambach, we have got to face this. We've got to find a pathway, God's pathway, for your healing to come out of this." God led us to a period of resting, a period of pulling apart and getting started on that pathway.

We did some tests on him. God instructed us to use a natural substance, found in plants, called coenzyme Q-10 (see Gen. 1:9-13). Then He instructed us through His Word regarding the foods to avoid, including fat (see Lev. 3:17; 7:23; 11:1-46).

He didn't tell us to put mud and saliva on Brother Shambach's heart (John 9), but He did instruct us to use a certain medication — a water pill (ACE drug) — and, of all things, to decrease *not* increase his water intake. Another medicine which is derived from a foxglove plant was used to regulate the heart rhythm.

After all these instructions, I can see us now sitting at a table in the clinic, our hands joined together praying the prayer of faith: The natural had joined the supernatural! After a five-month period of time, his heart had nearly doubled in its pumping capacity based on echocardiogram tests. "Praise God!" Brother Shambach was shouting when I told him that. We don't need a medical report to know that God is healing us. But thank God, He confirms His Word.

He confirmed and He answered the effectual prayers of the righteous man. We discerned God's pathway for Brother Shambach. I want him to share with you some of those lifestyle changes that he has made on a daily basis. This will help you see how a healing evangelist who believes in and ministers the supernatural healing power of God can follow God's pathway of healing for himself. It's been a challenge for him, but he is overcoming.

Bro. Shambach: Yes, and my wife helps me stay on the pathway that included a complete change of diet.

Dr. Cherry: It's not easy. But share with us what you do when you go into a restaurant. I mean, people need to know you don't just go in and order anything on the menu.

Bro. Shambach: I'll tell you what I do. I pull the waiter aside and say to him, "Before you talk to anybody, I want you to listen to me. I'm on a special diet. I can't have salt. I can't have butter. But I notice you have salmon on that menu, and I have a love affair with salmon. If you can broil that salmon with no salt, no butter, just do it. Give me a baked potato with no sour cream and no butter. And steam me some vegetables. Then we'll let the rest of them order. And if you can't do it this way, let me know now, and we'll go someplace else." And they do it.

Dr. Cherry: The righteous are as bold as a lion! Brother Shambach has taken charge of his health here boldly like a lion.

Bro. Shambach: I have. You have got to be a disciple following the pathway of healing that God has given you. And when it comes to the walking, I get up early in the morning and walk.

Dr. Cherry: How far do you walk?

Bro. Shambach: It's long! When I first came back, you told me not to walk at all. You wanted total rest then. And that was the toughest for me especially — total rest. And then after the first examination, you said, "I'm going to put you on a walking program for fifteen minutes daily for one week and then double it to thirty." And I took my wife out with me once. She said after one time around that shopping mall, "I'm going to wait here and have a cup of coffee. I'll catch you the next time around." But I get a good pace going, and I break a sweat. I have sweat running from my hair. Walking contributes to the regaining of the strength in that heart muscle.

Dr. Cherry: Let's go back to that restaurant. We talked about salmon. There have been some studies done around the world which show that there are groups of people, particularly Eskimos, who have nothing but salmon and cold water fish to eat. Salmon is a staple of their diet and other fish that fit in this same category are cod, herring and mackerel. These are probably the best fish that you can eat to reverse heart disease and to prevent heart disease if you don't have it. It's because of chemicals that we call omega-3 fatty acids that reduce the ability of platelets to stick together. When these platelets don't clump, heart disease drops.

Eskimos, particularly the Greenland Eskimos, the groups of people in the northern latitudes, have some of the lowest rates of heart disease in the world. And we find they eat large quantities of cold water fish. Scientists have now discovered that it's these omega-3 fatty acids that actually help to thin our blood. We need to find things that keep the blood flowing. When the blood stops flowing, life ceases.

The Bible tells us that the life is in the blood (Lev. 17:11). If you live in an industrialized country, chances are you have developed rough areas in many of your arteries that we call plaque, caused by cholesterol. As the blood flows through these arteries and encounters one of these rough areas, the platelets stick together and can form a blood clot. If the clot starts growing it can completely block the flow of blood, and anything downstream is going to die because the flow of oxygen is cut off. Life is in the blood. If the blood flow ceases, there is no life — there's death.

A heart attack which is caused by a clot can cause death to a segment of the heart muscle. If you lose too much heart muscle, it's all over. People who suffer heart attacks usually have damage to just one area of their heart.

Back to the salmon Brother Shambach was talking about. He's always been a big fan of salmon. But it's hard — many times when you order salmon in a restaurant it comes covered with butter and all kinds of fancy sauces that have fat in them. It's easy to just eat it as it comes — people take the easy way out and say, "Yes, salmon is great." You need salmon that's broiled but not covered with any butter, salt or sauces. Better yet, have it basted in olive oil; that can lower blood cholesterol levels.

Bro. Shambach: Here's what I tell waiters when I order. It's a little crude, but they get the point. I say, "Tell that chef back there to broil that salmon naked. I don't want anything on the thing." When you get down to the nitty-gritty, they can understand that. I say, "Bring me a lemon, and I'll squeeze that on it — lemon is good for you."

Dr. Cherry: How do you deal with the salt issue?

Bro. Shambach: Salt has not been a problem for me, Brother Cherry. Long ago my wife and I just tossed the salt shakers out.

Dr. Cherry: So you tell them not to salt the food.

Bro. Shambach: I say, "Steam it. Steam the vegetables. That's what I want."

Dr. Cherry: When you begin looking closely, salt is put into everything, isn't it? How do you avoid salt?

Bro. Shambach: I read labels. And I'll say, "Too much sodium in that." I like to go to the supermarket with my wife now, and I read labels. You can't get rid of all the sodium, but you get the lowest that you can find. For instance, tuna fish in the can. I found some good tuna fish that was low in salt. I also love onions. And they are good for you.

Dr. Cherry: That brings up an interesting subject. You know, onion is the cousin of garlic. Doesn't your wife use a lot of garlic?

Bro. Shambach: Yes. When she cooks the salmon she'll put the real cloves of garlic in there. And we both eat it, so nobody can tell who has garlic. She also hides garlic in chicken breasts. And there are many good vegetables. I like red peppers, instead of green peppers, cucumbers and tomatoes. And of course, I love my onions.

Dr. Cherry: So you like onions. I believe that God, as we seek Him, puts a taste in us for healthy things. Onions, it turns out, raise the level of the good cholesterol, HDL. This helps "pull" cholesterol from the artery walls.

Bro. Shambach: And I'm walking good right now. Don't leave out the exercise.

Dr. Cherry: Yes, exercise is part of it. We're making a doctor out of you! We put Brother Shambach on a garlic supplement, one-a-day equivalent to one clove a day, though he can still eat it in his food.

Bro. Shambach: But I had something else going for me. I had all these people praying for me, you see. You don't want to ever overlook that factor. I mean that is a tremendous factor. You know, a lot of preachers are so proud. When they have a problem, they don't want anybody to know about it because they want people to think they are superhuman. But, I mean, I believe in prayer.

I may get sick. And when I do, I'm coming right in front of that camera and say, "I want your prayers. Get on your face for me. I need all the prayers I can get." I need others to help me in my ministry. I can't do everything by myself. You said to me once, "Brother Shambach, Jesus couldn't do it all by Himself. He chose twelve men to help Him, and then He called seventy more. And if He couldn't do it alone, who do we think we are?" I want to thank God for Dr. Cherry insisting that I get rest and find people to help me and pray for me

Conclusion

So, you see, all of us — doctors, evangelists and everyone — need to follow God's pathway of healing. Just because God uses us as vessels of healing for others doesn't mean we can disregard His healing covenant for our own lives. His health laws are for everyone. Remember, Brother Shambach was not a young man when he had to change his eating habits and lifestyle. Yes, he knew God's Word, but in some areas of his life, he had to start seeking and obeying God's direction in a different walk in his healing.

I urge you to seek God's pathway of healing. Don't wait until an attack occurs as it did with Brother Shambach. He had to face surgery before changing his ways to line up with God's health laws for his life. You can start now. Follow God's pathway of healing for you. Allow Him to direct you through prayer. Seek Him for natural ways to enter into His healing covenant. I believe that everyone reading this book can discover God's pathway of healing and be healed! Start seeking His direction now. I'm praying for you!

Appendix A

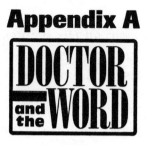

HEALING SCRIPTURES

The Bible says it is the spirit of man that will sustain him in his infirmity or disease (Prov. 18:14). You must continually hear and receive the Word of God so that the years of your life will be many (Prov. 4:10). The twenty-eight passages listed below are the basic verses God gave us for healing of the human body.* If you are fighting disease in your body, read each of them aloud daily. They will form the spiritual foundation for your healing.

1. If you will diligently hearken to the voice of the Lord your God and will do what is right in His

---

* All healing scriptures listed in the appendix are from the Amplified Bible.

sight, and will listen to and obey His commandments and keep all His statutes, I will put none
of the diseases upon you which I brought upon
the Egyptians, for I am the Lord Who heals you
(Ex. 15:26).

2. You shall serve the Lord your God; He shall
bless your bread and water, and I will take sickness from your midst (Ex. 23:25).

3 You shall be blessed above all peoples; there
shall not be male or female barren among you,
or among your cattle. And the Lord will take
away from you all sickness, and none of the
evil diseases of Egypt which you knew will He
put upon you, but will lay them upon all who
hate you (Deut. 7:14-15).

4. I call heaven and earth to witness this day
against you that I have set before you life and
death, the blessings and the curses; therefore
choose life, that you and your descendants may
live and may love the Lord your God, obey His
voice, and cling to Him. For He is your life and
the length of your days, that you may dwell in
the land which the Lord swore to give to your
fathers, to Abraham, Isaac, and Jacob (Deut.
30:19-20).

5. Blessed be the Lord, Who has given rest to His
people Israel, according to all that He promised.
Not one word has failed of all His good
promises which He promised through Moses
His servant (1 Kin. 8:56).

6. Because you have made the Lord your refuge,

and the Most High your dwelling place, there shall no evil befall you, nor any plague or calamity come near your tent...Because he has set his love upon Me, therefore will I deliver him; I will set him on high, because he knows and understands My name [has a personal knowledge of My mercy, love, and kindness — trusts and relies on Me, knowing I will never forsake him, no, never]. He shall call upon Me, and I will answer him; I will be with him in trouble. I will deliver him and honor him. With long life will I satisfy him and show him My salvation (Ps. 91:9-10,14-16)

7   Bless (affectionately, gratefully praise) the Lord, O my soul; and all that is [deepest] within me, bless His holy name! Bless (affectionately, gratefully praise) the Lord, O my soul, and forget not [one of] all His benefits — Who forgives [every one of] all your iniquities, Who heals [each one of] all your diseases, Who redeems your life from the pit and corruption, Who beautifies, dignifies, and crowns you with loving-kindness and tender mercy; Who satisfies your mouth [your necessity and desire at your personal age and situation] with good so that your youth, renewed, is like the eagle's [strong, overcoming, soaring]! (Ps. 103:1-5)

8. Then they cry to the Lord in their trouble, and He delivers them out of their distresses He sends forth His word and heals them and rescues them from the pit and destruction (Ps 107:19-20).

9. I shall not die but live, and shall declare the works and recount the illustrious acts of the Lord (Ps. 118:17).

10. My son, attend to my words; consent and submit to my sayings. Let them not depart from your sight; keep them in the center of your heart. For they are life to those who find them, healing and health to all their flesh. Keep and guard your heart with all vigilance and above all that you guard, for out of it flow the springs of life. Put away from you false and dishonest speech, and willful and contrary talk put far from you (Prov. 4:20-24).

11. Fear not [there is nothing to fear], for I am with you; do not look around you in terror and be dismayed, for I am your God. I will strengthen and harden you to difficulties, yes, I will help you; yes, I will hold you up and retain you with My [victorious] right hand of rightness and justice (Is. 41:10).

12. Surely He has borne our griefs (sicknesses, weaknesses, and distresses) and carried our sorrows and pains [of punishment], yet we [ignorantly] considered Him stricken, smitten, and afflicted by God [as if with leprosy] (Is. 53:4-5).

13. Then said the Lord to me, You have seen well, for I am alert and active, watching over My word to perform it (Jer. 1:12).

14. For I will restore health to you, and I will heal your wounds, says the Lord, because they have

called you an outcast, saying, This is Zion, whom no one seeks after and for whom no one cares! (Jer. 30:17).

15. Beat your plowshares into swords, and your pruning hooks into spears; let the weak say, I am strong [a warrior]! (Joel 3:10).

16. What do you devise and [how mad is your attempt to] plot against the Lord? He will make a full end [of Nineveh]; affliction [which My people shall suffer from Assyria] shall not rise up the second time (Nah. 1:9).

17. And behold, a leper came up to Him and, prostrating himself, worshiped Him, saying, Lord, if You are willing, You are able to cleanse me by curing me. And He reached out His hand and touched him, saying, I am willing; be cleansed by being cured. And instantly his leprosy was cured and cleansed (Matt. 8:2-3).

18. When evening came, they brought to Him many who were under the power of demons, and He drove out the spirits with a word and restored to health all who were sick. And thus He fulfilled what was spoken by the prophet Isaiah, He Himself took [in order to carry away] our weaknesses and infirmities and bore away our diseases (Matt. 8:16-17).

19. Truly I tell you, whatever you forbid and declare to be improper and unlawful on earth must be what is already forbidden in heaven, and whatever you permit and declare proper and lawful on earth must be what is already

permitted in heaven. Again I tell you, if two of you on earth agree (harmonize together, make a symphony together) about whatever [anything and everything] they may ask, it will come to pass and be done for them by My Father in heaven (Matt. 18:18-19).

20. And Jesus answered them, Truly I say to you, if you have faith (a firm relying trust) and do not doubt, you will not only do what has been done to the fig tree, but even if you say to this mountain, Be taken up and cast into the sea, it will be done (Matt. 21:21).

21. And Jesus, replying, said to them, Have faith in God [constantly]. Truly I tell you, whoever says to this mountain, Be lifted up and thrown into the sea! and does not doubt at all in his heart but believes that what he says will take place, it will be done for him. For this reason I am telling you, whatever you ask for in prayer, believe (trust and be confident) that it is granted to you, and you will [get it] (Mark 11:22-24).

22. Afterward He appeared to the Eleven [apostles themselves] as they reclined at table; and He reproved and reproached them for their unbelief (their lack of faith) and their hardness of heart, because they had refused to believe those who had seen Him and looked at Him attentively after He had risen [from death].

And He said to them, Go into all the world and preach and publish openly the good news (the Gospel) to every creature [of the whole human race].

He who believes [who adheres to and trusts

in and relies on the Gospel and Him Whom it sets forth] and is baptized will be saved [from the penalty of eternal death]; but he who does not believe [who does not adhere to and trust in and rely on the Gospel and Him Whom it sets forth] will be condemned.

And these attesting signs will accompany those who believe: in My name they will drive out demons; they will speak in new languages; they will pick up serpents; and [even] if they drink anything deadly, it will not hurt them; they will lay their hands on the sick, and they will get well (Mark 16:14-18).

23. Therefore, [inheriting] the promise is the outcome of faith and depends [entirely] on faith, in order that it might be given as an act of grace (unmerited favor), to make it stable and valid and guaranteed to all his descendants — not only to the devotees and adherents of the Law, but also to those who share the faith of Abraham, who is [thus] the father of us all.

As it is written, I have made you the father of many nations. [He was appointed our father] in the sight of God in Whom he believed, Who gives life to the dead and speaks of the nonexistent things that [He has foretold and promised] as if they [already] existed.

[For Abraham, human reason for] hope being gone, hoped in faith that he should become the father of many nations, as he had been promised, So [numberless] shall be your descendants be.

He did not weaken in faith when he considered the [utter] impotence of his own body, which was as good as dead because he was about a hundred years old, or [when he considered] the barrenness of Sarah's [deadened] womb.

No unbelief or distrust made him waver (doubtingly question) concerning the promise of God, but he grew strong and was empowered by faith as he gave praise and glory to God,

Fully satisfied and assured that God was able and mighty to keep His word and to do what He had promised (Rom. 4:16-21).

24. He personally bore our sins in His [own] body on the tree [as on an altar and offered Himself on it], that we might die (cease to exist) to sin and live to righteousness. By His wounds you have been healed (1 Pet. 2:24).

25. And, beloved, if our consciences (our hearts) do not accuse us [if they do not make us feel guilty and condemn us], we have confidence (complete assurance and boldness) before God, and we receive from Him whatever we ask, because we [watchfully] obey His orders [observe His suggestions and injunctions, follow His plan for us] and [habitually] practice what is pleasing to Him (1 John 3:21-22).

26. And this is the confidence (the assurance, the privilege of boldness) which we have in Him: [we are sure] that if we ask anything (make any request) according to His will (in agreement with His own plan), He listens to and hears us. And if (since) we [positively] know that He listens to us in whatever we ask, we also know

[with settled and absolute knowledge] that we have [granted us as our present possessions] the requests made of Him (1 John 5:14-15).

27. Beloved, I pray that you may prosper in every way and [that your body] may keep well, even as [I know] your soul keeps well and prospers (3 John 2).

28. And they have overcome (conquered) him by means of the blood of the Lamb and by the utterance of their testimony, for they did not love and cling to life even when faced with death [holding their lives cheap till they had to die for their witnessing] (Rev. 12:11).

Subject Index

About the Author

Dr. Cherry and his wife, Linda, conduct a weekly television program, *The Doctor and the Word,* aired over Trinity Broadcasting Network (TBN) stations, TBN affiliate stations and local stations that carry TBN programming. On this program, which is based on actual case studies of patients from their clinic, Dr. Cherry and his wife discuss the biblical perspective of healing and nutrition, showing that healing can come supernaturally and through the use of natural substances and treatment.

Dr. Cherry is the founder and director of the R. B. Cherry Clinic for Preventive Medicine in Houston, Texas. The clinic evaluates patients to detect the presence or absence of disease in various body systems. Particular attention is focused on major diseases such as heart and vascular disease and cancer. After thorough testing, detailed recommendations are given for the treatment of existing illness and the elimination of potential health problems. Each patient receives individualized nutrition and exercise programs as well as guidance in a program of supplemental natural substances. These programs are developed after the patient's test results have been reviewed by Dr. Cherry.

If you would like further information about the clinic, or wish to contact Dr. Cherry directly, please write:

Dr. R. B. Cherry
The R. B. Cherry Clinic for Preventive Medicine
One West Loop South, Suite 702
Houston, TX 77027
Phone: 713-961-0423

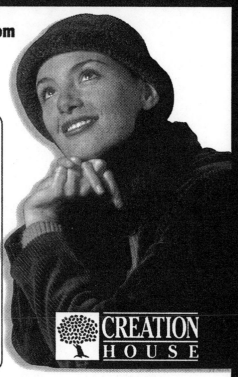